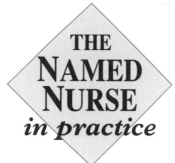

THE NAMED NURSE
in practice

Rosie Dargan

MPhil, BA(Hons), RGN

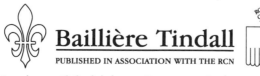

Baillière Tindall

PUBLISHED IN ASSOCIATION WITH THE RCN

London • Philadelphia • Toronto • Sydney • Tokyo

Baillière Tindall   24–28 Oval Road
London NW1 7DX

The Curtis Center
Independence Square West
Philadelphia, PA 19106-3399, USA

Harcourt Brace & Company
55 Horner Avenue
Toronto, Ontario, M8Z 4X6, Canada

Harcourt Brace & Company, Australia
30–52 Smidmore Street
Marrickville
NSW 2204, Australia

Harcourt Brace & Company, Japan
Ichibancho Central Building
22–1 Ichibancho
Chiyoda-ku, Tokyo 102, Japan

A catalogue record for this book is available from the British Library

ISBN 1-873853-37-8

Typeset by Florencetype Ltd, Stoodleigh, Devon
Printed and bound in Great Britain by WBC Book Manufacturers,
Bridgend, Glamorgan

To Dallan and Anna

Contents

Foreword

When the various Patient's Charters emerged the response among nurses was along a continuum – from apathy to enthusiasm. For many nurses it was not a new idea – those who had been practising primary nursing, or managing their own case loads in the community, could justifiably say that it was what they were doing anyway. Yet for many, especially those in the hospital setting, developing a named nurse approach has proved highly problematic. Caught up in the busy world of work, with elbows to the wheel and noses to the grindstone, it can be very difficult to look up and see a vision of how things might be done differently. It also needs to be remembered that the responsibility for successful implementation does not rest with nurses alone, but with policy makers, managers, teachers and others who support the caring environment.

Inevitably there has also been a focus of concern about the workings of named nursing – what happens if the nurse goes off sick, how does it work on night duty, what about accountability? Although the Department of Health published detailed guidance, to which Rosie refers in this book, this was quickly taken up and there has been remarkably little published on the theme since that time – perhaps somewhat surprisingly in view of the major significance of this policy. I therefore welcome this text as a timely and much needed addition to the literature. It is right that nurses should be concerned with the practicalities, not just because it is a national policy, nor because patients will expect it, nor because it places nursing as central to healthcare (it is the first time in history that any government, anywhere, has made a public statement to its population about an entitlement to nursing), it is all of these and more, but because the intention is to make care better for patients. Although it has become a national policy, we should not lose sight of the fact that this initiative is very much driven by nurses in practice and rooted in nursing practice.

Furthermore, named nursing is not just about getting the organi-sational patterns right, but about transforming the nature of the nurse–patient relationship, about nourishing the context in which creative, compassionate caring can emerge to help and heal another human being. I hope very much that nurses will use this book as an aide in turning a vision into reality.

Professor Stephen G Wright

MBE, RGN, DipN, RCNT, DANS, RNT, MSc(Nursing), MHSM, FRCN

Preface

WHAT DOES IT MEAN TO BE A NAMED NURSE?

The Charter Standard is that you should have a named, qualified nurse, midwife or health visitor who will be responsible for your nursing or midwifery care.
(Charter Statement No. 8, Department of Health 1991)

The Patient's Charter promised the British public a 'named nurse'. However, the allocation of a named nurse to a patient does not automatically change the method of care management, the bedside attitude, the standard of care provision, or the power of the patient to control his environment.

It is not enough to say that named nursing means just what it says. What does it say? What are the implications of being a named nurse for the nurse, the patient, and the nursing team? What is the role of the ward manager in named nursing? What does named nursing offer the nurse today who must face the uncertainty of the future?

The author has used the generally accepted simplification of referring to all patients as he and all nurses as she. No insult is intended and the weakness of the above method is recognised.

Acknowledgements

During the writing of this book I seem to have taken advantage of all of my friends in one way or another and I am grateful for the opportunity to thank you all for your support.

In this regard I would like to mention Claire, my friend, typist and advisor, you know how necessary you were; and Rosemarie Buchanan for your constant encouragement and guidance.

All of the staff at Queens University Medical Library were supportive above and beyond the call of duty and among this group of friends Patricia Watt deserves special acknowledgement.

I would also like to express my individual thanks to Gerry, Maura, Brenda, Mary and Sean.

Introduction

The health care environment is changing rapidly. Such a pace of change inevitably brings casualties – either those who cannot keep up with the change, or those who fail to fit into the new structure.

As an integral part of the health care environment, the nursing profession incurs the effects of this change process. At the forefront are nurses breaking new ground, and perhaps changing the face of nursing forever, while for the majority of nurses the reality is that the practice of nursing continues relatively unchanged (Pearson 1992), and they struggle within a tightly structured routine to keep up to date on nursing trends and theory and to close the yawning gap between the practice of nursing and nursing research.

This book is designed to be a tool to assist those nurses who wish to close that gap, to keep up with the changes, and to build into their practice sufficient flexibility so that they may find a place to nurse within whatever new structures are created. It addresses the frustration created by the knowledge that while the vestiges of Victorian subservience still linger, the nurse leaders of tomorrow will be looking for autonomous, self-motivated, research-oriented practitioners to achieve their goals. The book will assist nurses wishing to invest in their future by practising flexibility and self-directed nursing.

Although named nursing was given its formal title when John Major introduced the concept into *The Patient's Charter* in 1991 (Department of Health 1991), some would argue that it had been a part of nursing methodology long before this (Hancock 1992a; Wright 1992) in the practice of midwives and community nurses, and in the hospital setting, as an aspect of the primary nursing model of care.

Named nursing therefore is not a revolutionary new idea for the nursing profession, requiring years of analysis or debate. In Hancock's (1992a) view the ground has already been well prepared for the named nurse idea, and both Hancock (1992a) and Wright (1993) recognise not only the simplicity of the concept, but also that putting it into practice should require neither massive resources nor much upheaval.

The Patient's Charter states that each patient is entitled to a named nurse. But since it failed to specify the duties of care incumbent on that 'named nurse', or the benefits to be gained by a patient who has a named nurse, implementing the charter standard can prove difficult in the absence of specific guidelines.

When the term was coined, for many nurses it seemed familiar, and reminiscent of primary nursing, but somehow different. Is it a watered-down version of primary nursing? If the answer to this is yes, then primary nursing is superior, and the patient who is allocated to a 'named nurse' rather than a 'primary nurse' would be losing out.

For named nursing to succeed, it should be seen as separate and distinct from primary nursing while accepting its origins in the primary nursing model of care.

The following text offers a structure for the named nurse, and for the ward or unit which practises named nursing. It offers guidance for clinical supervision for the ward manager, and is also designed as a tool to assist the practising nurse in coping with the inevitable changes ahead, and to allow her to control the pace of change at practice level. One of these changes is that the named nurse and the key worker concepts are interchangeable, even within hospitals. In addressing this goal, the practice discussions should become multidisciplinary (see Chapter 4). The structure also offers a means for the patient to participate in his care via both the structured discussions and the patient questionnaire (see Chapter 2). This aspect of the named nursing structure acknowledges the increasing requirement for the patient to be given the opportunity to have a more specific voice in his care both with regard to informed choices, and consumer satisfaction indices.

1
Background
Discussions

The theory-practice gap – Where we are today –
Structure for successful change – The four structures for
change – Communication made visible – What will
tomorrow bring? – Designed to fit in

THE THEORY-PRACTICE GAP

One of the difficulties for the nursing profession at the end of the
20th century is the enormity of the gap between the profession's
theorists and its practitioners. This gap has persisted for probably
the whole of the 20th century (Kramer 1974; Bendall 1975;
Wright 1986; Pearson 1988; Castledine 1993), and now, in the
approach to the 21st century, nurse education is being taught in
higher education venues, creating what Castledine (1993) termed
a 'new urgency' in facing the reality of knowledge-based nursing
practice.

The lack of commitment to nursing practice by senior members
of our profession (Castledine 1993) is probably one of the main
reasons that, regardless of the volumes of research findings and
models of care, at the bedside, very little real change can be identified (Pearson 1988; Wright 1990; Astley 1992). Change theories
abound, but almost invariably the change is initiated from the top
down, rather than the bottom up. Wright (1986) blames the failure
to implement change on 'the **unstructured approach** adopted
by the innovators' (author's emphasis), and Wright (1986) and
Cole (1993) identify the lack of ownership permitted to those
who are doing the work. 'By owning the change, the staff come
to feel it is their decision. It is their property. We tend to cherish,
care for, and preserve those things we ourselves have created'

(Wright 1986). In the context of Lewin's (1947) view of change as unfreezing and refreezing, Wright (1986) says 'in order to "unfreeze" existing norms and "move" staff to "refreeze" into new norms, a tool to do the job is required'.

However we are all so much creatures of habit that unless we can find a new routine fairly quickly, we are liable collectively, to revert to the tried and trusted method of getting the work done.

Nurse leaders are unanimous (Wright 1991) in their call for a planned approach to change (Pearson 1985; Pearson and Vaughan 1986; Turrell 1986; Salvage 1988; Wright 1989).

WHERE WE ARE TODAY

The secret to success in changing anything is for the designer of the changes to have a clear concept of the reality of the situation before the change. It is not enough to have a vision of where we are going. We must equally have a vision of where we are coming from. It is necessary to be clear about not only **what** nursing is and what it is not, but **where** nursing is and where it is not.

The library shelves are full of books on how nursing care should be delivered. However, in order to bring in real, lasting change, it is necessary to begin the change from the reality of how the nurse at the bedside is practising today. This, in many situations, can still be identified as **routine-focused**, **system-focused** nursing (Pearson 1992). Recognising all the constraints and force fields which inhibit a change to patient-focused care is the first step in the change process.

STRUCTURE FOR SUCCESSFUL CHANGE

The second step is to provide a structure for change which can fit into current work practices. This structure should ideally require little effort to implement and should have potential for continuous development, plus sufficient flexibility to facilitate growth at different rates to suit individual and collective needs.

The strategy for change in the named nurse programme is based on the fact that change has already been decreed – every patient in Britain is now entitled to a named nurse as a result of *The Patient's Charter* (Department of Health 1991). This is a top-down approach to change and nursing has in the past managed to resist this approach quite successfully.

THE FOUR STRUCTURES FOR CHANGE

The named nurse programme is a planned strategy using a bottom-up approach (see Figure 1.1). It offers a package of four separate structures which, when interlinked and used productively, are mutually supportive in achieving the following objectives:

■ Goal-directed patient/nurse communication;

■ Nursing coordination of patient care;

■ Informed participation of patients in their care;

■ Nurse development;

■ Practice/research updating;

■ Practice development;

■ Clinical supervision;

■ Regular clinical audit;

■ Managerial monitoring of care planning;

■ Improved patient care management;

■ Forum for consumer opinion on care;

■ Opportunity for multidisciplinary input into change processes.

These four structures are subdivided into two for the nurse/patient, and two for the nurse manager. The first takes the form of goal-directed meetings with the patient. These are described in Chapter 2. The purpose of these meetings is to guide the nurse and the patient towards goal achievement through patient empowerment.

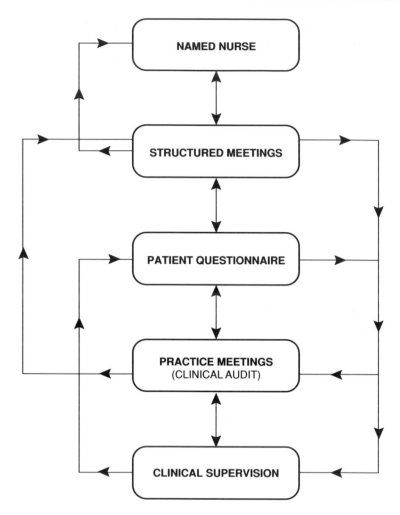

Figure 1.1   The named nursing programme with feedback loops.

The second is a patient questionnaire, also discussed in Chapter 2. This acts not only as a means of empowerment for the patient by giving him a voice, but also provides a self-evaluation tool for the nurse, in that it asks for the patient's views of his named nurse, and the responses are addressed to the named nurse personally.

The third and fourth structures involve the ward manager as supporter of the named nurse. Her input is to:

1. conduct monthly practice meetings which will foster continually up-dated research-based nursing practice and act as a clinical audit using Salvage's (1990) description as a cycle of activity which requires the nurse to 'look at what you are currently doing, determine what you should be doing and take action to close the gap between the real and the ideal'

2. support the named nurse by taking on the role of clinical supervisor. Chapter 4 describes a means of doing this using the practice meetings as guidelines and the care plans as indicators.

These structures are designed to empower the nursing staff to take control of the nursing practice in their area, to implement change – at their own pace – and to do this starting from where they are today.

Although it is designed as a bottom-up approach to change it is essential that the management executive fully understand the concept of the named nurse and how to monitor its effectiveness. Therefore, Chapter 6 addresses the input required from senior management, and the rewards to be gained by the hospital generally.

COMMUNICATION MADE VISIBLE

Although the named nursing programme fits into the highly visible, frequently rewarded, nurse and system-oriented task-ridden routine of the daily work schedule, it is designed to dismantle ineffective routines and focus nursing practice on individual patient needs, and client-oriented low-visibility tasks. Bradley and Edinberg (1990) differentiate between the high visibility of physiological functions which 'are easily broken down into steps, and require a high degree of psychomotor manual skill. At a less obvious level, they are easily routinised and are staff-centred' and low-visibility tasks which 'are not easily seen by others, are usually related to psychological actions, require cognitive or affective skills as opposed to psychomotor skills, and cannot usually be broken down into identifiable steps . . . They are also "client-oriented" . . .'.

Providing a structure for named nursing turns a low visibility task (interpersonal communication) into a high visibility task thus giving it official credibility in the daily routine, and placing it in an arena for reward within the hospital setting. It also addresses the fact that approximately 70% of all consumer complaints involve poor communication in some form or other (Department of Health 1994a).

How does the consumer, in the form of the patient, measure the quality of the service he receives? With whom does he communicate for the majority of the time he spends in hospital? **The nurse is the most visible interpretation of hospital care, and her communication skills may be the measure by which patients and relatives interpret the quality of care provided**.

WHAT WILL TOMORROW BRING?

Professional nursing will soon have to fight to retain an integral role in the future health care arena where it is envisaged that trackless image-guided surgery can be performed thousands of miles away from the treated patient (Wyke 1994). This is not fantasy! Already ROBODOC, a surgical robot designed to perform surgery, and purported to be 20 times more accurate than a human doctor, concluded its clinical trials by 1995 (Wyke 1994). This, however, is only one of the mind-blowing computerised devices for patient-care management planned to be operational by the year 2010.

Will the nurse of tomorrow be confined to being a bedside computer technician?

One of roles of the nurse in the future will be to protect and safeguard the interpersonal aspect of patient management. The named nurse programme, in providing a structured relationship with the patient, assists the nurse in this goal.

However, before the nurse can change the way she practises, she needs to be able to interpret and recognise her own very personal intuitive theories and models by which she practises. Until the nurse can feel sufficiently free within her working environment to reflect on her practice she will have difficulty identifying flaws or areas for improvement.

Practice meetings offer an opportunity for reflection and interpretation both for individual nurses and for the nursing staff as a group. This bottom-up mode of change has been recommended. The chances of the change surviving 'are better if it is rooted in the system as a regular working situation' (Ottoway 1976). The busy practice nurse however may also need a guide as to how to bring about the changes that she wants. She may need a structure (Pearson 1985; Pearson and Vaughan 1986; Turrell 1986; Salvage 1988; Wright 1989, 1991), not just a structure which guides her actions, but one which promotes professional growth, ongoing value analysis, practice effectiveness appraisal, method analysis and personal and group development.

DESIGNED TO FIT IN

The named nurse programme is designed to 'fit in' to whatever structure is in place. It does not demand radical change for initial implementation. However it sets the agenda for continuing change controlled by those who will be implementing that change.

Luin (1947) emphasised in his normative–re-educative model of change, the need not only for 'new motoric actions', or a new structure of behaviour, but also the need for re-education as a means for refreezing that behaviour. The new structure alone will not necessarily produce lasting change unless the practitioners' attitudes to their practice are also given room to develop, as Lawler (1991) says about expert practitioners, 'it is not what they do but "how" they do it'. Attitudes and developmental processes are given scope in the practice meeting, the self-evaluation tool and the clinical supervision programme. These structures should also highlight which skills are needed to implement new concepts, and will encourage training to follow change as Ottoway (1976) recommends.

2

A Structured Role for the Named Nurse

Choosing to change – Structure as empowerment tool – More than a name – The core of named nursing – What does a named nurse do? – First meeting structure – Intermediate meetings structure – Final or discharge meeting structure – The nurse's personal card – The named nurse's personal evaluation tool

CHOOSING TO CHANGE

In choosing to be a named nurse have no doubt about the choice you are making. Nursing today is in a position to be more powerful than ever before, because the named nurse standard in *The Patient's Charter* has given public credence to the nursing profession to provide an autonomous, self-directed, patient-focused relationship with the patient (see Chapter 5 for discussions on power). So choose between inertia and action (see Figure 2.1).

If the nurse at the bedside does not begin to take some control of her profession now, the opportunity may become increasingly difficult as the boundaries become blurred in the future.

As in most organisations, (Peters 1989) the principal enemy in nursing is **inertia**, and those nurses who are not progressing professionally, do not stand still. If you are not progressing, you are regressing. Power, according to Bailey and Claus (1975) requires three underlying factors: strength, energy and action.

The hospital system, with its rigid bureaucracy, has unwittingly placed a straightjacket on the individual professional development needs of the nurse, forcing her to conform to the norm, to the mediocrity of stability. The implementation of a structured named

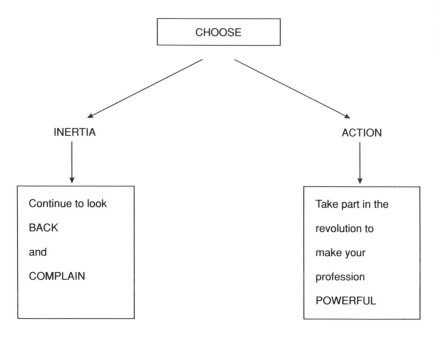

Figure 2.1   Choose: inertia *vs* action.

nursing programme frees the individual practitioner to develop within any system, by giving her structured time, the opportunity for feedback both from the patient and the ward manager, and a forum specifically to promote continued questioning, evaluating and improving nursing practice.

The structure is designed to give the named nurse 'time' with her patients which the Audit Commission (1992) recommends should be a 'necessary part of the nurse's day'.

STRUCTURE AS EMPOWERMENT TOOL

However, it is not enough to recommend making time for patients within a highly structured environment. It must be

STRUCTURED TIME

to ensure that it successfully competes with so many traditional/ structured forces demanding priority throughout the day.

> STRUCTURE

according to Peter Druker (1967) is the

> TOOL

you use to achieve your

> GOALS AND OBJECTIVES

The named nurse programme, therefore, by providing a structure for implementing named nursing, acts as a tool to enable the goals and objectives of named nursing to be achieved. The simplicity of the structure reduces anxiety in implementation. Burnard (1989) sums it up: 'we are frightened by what we do not understand. Such fear and lack of clarity often leads in turn to inaction'.

Named nursing is a very

> SIMPLE

concept but its very simplicity belies its

> POWER.

It empowers the nurse, the patient, and the nursing team.

The structured named nurse programme offers a **base** from which to build, and, in the final chapter, there are suggestions on how to improve the basic structure. This structure enables named nursing to succeed, regardless of the management style currently in use.

Once you decide to start –

S T A R T   T O D A Y .

Named nursing offers you the power to change the way you practise forever. So take possession of that power, and start the ball rolling. A ball which will still be rolling after you retire, even if, by then, it has altered its shape somewhat.

You take control

You start it

You make it happen

This does not mean that your nursing practice today is inadequate. Many nurse writers recognise that frequently neither nurses nor others value the work that nurses do (Manthey 1980; Audit Commission 1991; Hancock 1992b; Wright 1993).

However 'such is the pace and volume of change in health care these days that the idea of nursing having to fight for its rightful place at the forefront of patient care is not a controversial one' (Gilbert 1994).

Nurses are continually striving to improve both the care they provide to their patients, and the environment within which that care is provided.

MORE THAN A NAME

Many nurses believe that they are practising named nursing, and will display the visible signs of the named nurse practice of care. For example:

■ Boards are clearly visible at the entrance to or in a dominant area on the ward with lists of patient's names, consultant's names, and nurse's names.

■ A card is attached to the head of the bed with the consultant's name and the nurse's name clearly written.

■ Patients are questioned on a regular basis as to the name of their nurse, and prompted with a name if they can't remember.

The visible signs are indeed present, but scrape a little deeper ... As Eileen Brady (1992) asks, after her experience of named nursing with a nurse called Bernie, 'Where is the assessment and planning ... Where is the skilled counselling of the patient ... where is Bernie?'.

Brady goes on to say 'I feel we are giving the profession a bad name and could be accused of hypocrisy by pretending to deliver what we cannot or do not intend to offer our patients .... Patients need good quality care given by good nurses, not a name on a bit of card attached to the top of the bed'.

THE CORE OF NAMED NURSING

The core of named nursing is more than just the visible signs of the nurse's name at the bed, on the notice boards, and/or on the patient's charts. The core of named nursing is that

THE NAMED NURSE

COORDINATES

THE PATIENT'S

CARE

and

THE PATIENT GIVES

HIS INFORMED

CONSENT TO THAT

CARE.

The Audit Commission (1991) recognises that nurses are best placed to 'co-ordinate other professionals' work with the patient'.

From the patient's point of view the core of named nursing is potential empowerment and control of decisions as a result of the content and quality of the nurse–patient meetings.

From Florence Nightingale through to the Audit Commission Report (1991) the patient/nurse relationship is recognised as the core of nursing. The Audit Commission (1991) even quotes Nightingale who says that 'it is better to know the patient in a certain condition than the condition from which the patient may suffer'.

From these meetings the patient should be empowered to voice his opinions and his choices and to see these affecting the decisions on his care management.

The healing effect of activities such as information giving is well recognised in nursing (Hayward 1975; Wilson-Barnett 1978, 1988; Davies 1985; Thompson 1989; Hockey 1991) and McMahon (1991) have traced the concept back to Nightingale (1859) with the quote that 'apprehension, uncertainty, waiting, expectation, fear of surprise, do a patient more harm than any exertion'.

The following pages offer a guide to the patient–nurse meetings and a sample record sheet for the care plan. The first meeting is specific in format, as is the final or discharge meeting. Each intermediate meeting may vary depending on patient needs, but so long as a recognised format is practised the system should succeed.

WHAT DOES A NAMED NURSE DO?

To be a patient's named nurse you must:

1. **Be aware** of your limits of freedom of choice in accepting patients (see Chapter 3).

2. **Conduct** your first meeting with your patient within 24 hours of admission.

3. **The meeting may be** with the patient, or the carer/relatives, or both together.

4. **It would be ideal** if you were the patient's first point of contact on admission to the unit.

5. **After the first meeting** you must either

   ■ accept the nursing care plan and update it as necessary
   ■ amend the nursing care plan
   ■ write an appropriate nursing care plan
   ■ communicate any changes in nursing plans to the patient.

6. **Sign and date** your authorisation of he patient's nursing plan of care.

7. **You must be able** to support your nursing care plans with relevant, continually updated practice-based research recommendations (Lewis and Batey 1982; Vaughan and Pillmoor 1989) (see Chapter 4 on practice meetings).

8. **Set** and **record** realistic measurable goals and target dates which are, if possible, mutually agreed between the patient and yourself.

9. **Coordinate** the patient's care – within the accepted limits of multidisciplinary support practices in the area.

10. **State** on the plan the pre-requisites for discharge. (Ref: multi-disciplinary team decision).

11. **Participate** in the nursing care of your patients according to the current ward management methodology.

12. **Evaluate** the patient's nursing care plan after each structured meeting – and **re-sign** and **re-date**. When changes are made to the care plan these must be re-authorised, signed and dated within 72 hours at the latest (the 72 hours allows for the named nurse's days off, and is the *only* time when the 72 hour gap should exist).

13. **Have a structured meeting** at agreed times with each patient **at least** every two days but preferably more often. (This will depend on the individual patient's needs and the nurse's duty rota.)

14. **Record** each meeting on the named nurse record sheet (see Figure 2.2), or the care plan.

Named Nurse Record Sheet

Name: Address:
(or addressograph label)

D.O.B.:

Hospital no.:

Admissions summary:

Projected outcomes of care:

Patient questionnaire given: Date:

Multidisciplinary contacts:
(including community contacts)

Date:	Name:	Purpose:

Figure 2.2 The named nurse record sheet.

Named Nurse Record Sheet Patient/nurse meetings		
Dates:	Comments:	Signature:

Figure 2.2   (continued).

No structure, or text, or hospital policy will turn a nurse who is just technically competent into a therapeutic nurse. Each named nurse will approach her patient with her own particular skills and inadequacies. The long-term goal for the named nurse is to develop self-awareness from which she can map her journey of **becoming** rather than just **being**. It might be useful to find a good role model – how do you identify one? I have always used the yardstick – 'would I like her to nurse my mother?'. While this is simplistic it is a base for recognising a therapeutic nurse in action.

Communication with the patient is the core of the named nurse programme, but communication with a purpose. The purpose is specific to his need for care/cure. Management of the care plan is a written extension of the structured communication, and promotes goal-oriented nursing care. Therefore, if a care plan is required, the named nurse is responsible for that plan within the accepted limits mentioned above.

FIRST MEETING STRUCTURE

Being admitted to hospital can be a traumatic event. The memories and effects of this event may remain with the patient until his death. These events are more memorable than, for example, a splendid vacation. So do not underestimate the effects of your words and actions during this very vulnerable time for your patients.

TIME: Allow at least 15 mins.

1. **Introduction**. Develop an active listening approach. Remember – patients are rarely sufficiently empowered to ask the questions that they really want to ask.

2. **Assess** the patient's motivation and ability to co-operate.

3. **Inform** the patient that as his named nurse you will discuss his care with him on a regular basis.

4. **Explain** that as the named nurse you will be coordinating his nursing care plan and will guide him through his care whilst he is in the unit.

5. **Discuss** the patient-centred goals to be set, the care plan, and the dates for evaluation, including self-care and education goals.

6. **Describe** as honestly and sensitively as possible, the projected outcomes within agreed multidisciplinary guidelines and decisions.

7. **Explain** all medical interventions within agreed multidisciplinary guidelines.

8. **Determine** the patient's understanding of his reasons for hospitalisation, and his experiences since admission.

9. **Check** that nursing and medical notes correlate with this.

10. **Record** his level of understanding of his condition and of the agreed plans for his care.

11. **Encourage** him to question and give him time to communicate, remembering that illness is in itself disempowering.

12. **Plan** the patient's discharge with him, including a target discharge date, if this is a realistic option, recognising the benefits of early discharge planning on length of stay and reduced rates of re-hospitalisation (Naylor 1990; Naylor and Shaid 1991).

13. **Plan** to meet carers/relatives, as appropriate.

14. **Write** the date and time of the next meeting with him on your personal card and leave it on his locker.

15. **Authorise** his care plan. Sign and date it.

16. **Contact** multidisciplinary team members as appropriate.

17. **Communicate** with relevant nursing staff.

18. **Record** your meeting on the Meetings Record Sheet (Figure 2.2) or in the care plan.

INTERMEDIATE MEETINGS STRUCTURE

TIME: allow approximately 10 mins.

1. **Greet** the patient in a manner which facilitates empowerment.

2. **Remind** the patient that this meeting is to discuss his plan of care and how he **feels** about it – this is **his time**.

3. **Assess** the patient's perception of his plan of care and of his progress.

4. **Encourage** him to ask questions, express emotions, and to voice any fears or apprehensions he may have.

5. **Listen** actively, ensuring that your sitting position is appropriate. 'To truly listen to another person is perhaps the most caring action of all' (Burnard 1989).

6. **Answer** questions as honestly as possible.

7. **Assess** his progress with a patient-centred goal-oriented structure.

8. **Modify** the care plan with him as required.

9. **Discuss** the plans for discharge, if appropriate, and continuity of goals to be achieved outside the hospital setting.

10. **Write** the time and date of the next meeting on the named nurse personal card (see below).

11. **Record** contents of meeting. Sign and date the record.

12. **Communicate** any changes to relevant members of staff.

FINAL OR DISCHARGE MEETING STRUCTURE

TIME: allow approximately 15 mins.

1. **Greet** the patient in a manner which facilitates empowerment.

2. **Encourage** the patient to question or seek clarification of any aspects of his care or condition – remind him that this is **his time**.

3. **Discuss** the goals set at the other meetings and whether or not they have been achieved.

4. **Reinforce** any continuity of goals to be achieved outside the hospital setting.

5. **Record** his condition on discharge as compared with **your** care plan projections. Sign and date.

6. **Check** home support.

7. **Explain** all community care supports which he may require, which may include statutory, voluntary and independent agencies.

8. **Arrange** outpatient appointment **or** explain how this will happen.

9. **Reinforce** previous health and medication advice, both verbally and in writing.

10. **Finalise** transport arrangements.

11. **Give** him a patient questionnaire and an envelope addressed to you. Explain that this is a self-evaluation tool for your own personal use.

12. **Encourage** him to return the questionnaire.

The final meeting is the only meeting which, in some situations, may need to be delegated to another member of staff. Discharge can happen fairly suddenly in hospital and if a patient is told that he can go home today, the named nurse may not be available. The duty nurse then conducts the final or discharge meeting and makes a record to that effect. However, this is not satisfactory either for the patient, the named nurse, or the nurse performing the discharge. The goal is for the named nurse to discharge her patients, communicate with the relevant community personnel, and to provide each patient with written information on a standard form. Attaining that goal might be one of the topics discussed in the practice meetings.

THE NURSE'S PERSONAL CARD

Another useful tool is a personal card which you may give to your patient on first meeting.

This can be a card for use by all named nurses on the ward with blank spaces for the patient's name, the nurse's name and the date and times of each meeting. Figure 2.3 is a sample which can be photocopied and used on the ward.

You may wish to personalise it further by selecting your own colour of paper, or photocopying a small photograph of yourself in the top right-hand corner, or both. In some situations a re-usable card with washable ink pens might be appropriate.

THE NAMED NURSE'S PERSONAL EVALUATION TOOL

The objective of the patient questionnaire is twofold. It offers an opportunity for the patient to comment on his care, and by reflecting on the patient's comments, the nurse can use it as a means of personal evaluation. Good nursing care is often not recognised or acknowledged and the nurse has no record of her performance.

Name:		
Ward:		small photograph
(or addressograph label)		
Nurse's name:		

Date of meeting:	Time of meeting:	Signature

Name:		
Ward:		small photograph
(or addressograph label)		
Nurse's name:		

Date of meeting:	Time of meeting:	Signature

Figure 2.3 Nurse's personal card.

Name of hospital:

Address of hospital:

Name: Address:
(or Addressograph Label)

Name of ward(s):

When were you in this hospital?

       From: To:

Did you benefit from having a named nurse?   Yes   No
Please comment   ☐   ☐

Have you any suggestions on how I could have been more supportive?
Please comment

Figure 2.4   Sample patient questionnaire.

Self-evaluation, as a method of development enables the nurse to assess her practice and skills, and to reflect on the nursing care given. **The patient, in his own way, has more information about you as a nurse than has your line manager.** You should take advantage of this. Figure 2.4 is a sample questionnaire which may be given to the patient with an envelope for return addressed to **you** as his named nurse. Modify this to suit yourself, or write your own questionnaire.

The patient questionnaire may be presented to the patient at any time during his care, for example it may be:

■ Posted out to him prior to his admission;

■ Given to him on admission;

■ Presented at the first meeting, or at an intermediate meeting, or just prior to discharge;

■ A carer/relative may be the most appropriate person to receive the questionnaire.

Ask the patient to return this to you and use the comments as a means of enhancing self-awareness, as an opportunity for improving the care you give, and as a means of understanding patients' needs.

Explain to the patient that he may return the questionnaire either to you or the ward manager. The purpose of providing this option is to further enhance the patient's sense of involvement. It provides another avenue for the patient to exercise empowerment. If the patient wishes to make a complaint he can choose whether this should be addressed to you personally, or to the ward manager. Do not be frightened of this method of evaluation. It should only confirm your records of the patient/nurse meetings. (See Chapter 3 on the management of complaints.)

3

Ward Management of the Named Nurse Programme

Who can be a named nurse? – Named nursing and freedom to refuse – Allocation of nurses to patients – Who decides? – The question of overall responsibility – To associate or not to associate – Transfers to and from other wards – Staff absences – Personality preferences – Patient access to nurse duty rotas – Ward management of patient questionnaire responses – Managing complaints – Summary

In the previous chapter, staff nurses wishing to be more focused in their named nurse role were encouraged to start using the meeting structure with patients as a first step in the named nurse programme.

This chapter recognises that implementing the named nurse programme on a ward will raise some questions about ward management. The main issue involved in the administration of this programme in a ward context are discussed.

WHO CAN BE A NAMED NURSE?

To be a named nurse requires the knowledge and skill of a qualified first level nurse. So from the individual worker's stand-point the minimum requirement is first level registration.

From the patient's vantage point, the nurse should not only be knowledgeable and skilled, but also, and this is perhaps the most important requirement for the patient, she should **be there**.

So, in deciding who should be named, it is not enough to say either that all registered nurses are entitled to be named, or that only those nurses who work full-time on day duty should be allocated to patients.

If you examine the pattern of patient's stay the decision on suitability of part-time, casual, or night-duty staff as named nurses will be clarified. The question is simply – will the nurse be there for the majority of the patient's stay?

NAMED NURSING AND FREEDOM TO REFUSE

The Royal College of Nursing in their book *Refusal to Nurse, Guidance for Nurses* (1993) has provided guidance to nurses on circumstances in which a nurse may refuse to care for a patient. Apart from the Abortion Act (1967) and the Human Fertilisation and Embryology Act (1990), the circumstances cited are:

1. 'When it is believed that the nurse lacks the competence to provide care. Nurses therefore need to have due regard for maintaining professional competence in their area of work and need to ensure that their managers are aware of any limitations to practice,

2. When the patient is a relative or friend'.

It refers to the UKCC's *Code of Professional Conduct* (1992) which is very clear on the point that nurses have no right to be selective about patients.

However, 'caring for a patient', and 'being a named nurse for a patient' are slightly different and Tingle (1993) discusses the legal aspects of exercising choice in the practice of named nursing.

In reality this exercising of freedom will happen very rarely if the system is properly set up. However it is essential that the named nurse is aware of her freedom to exercise choice as a legal requirement. There are three main reasons for this necessity.

1. Some nurses may feel that they are not ready to be named nurses. If this is the case and they voice their reticence to the ward manager, the responsibility is then placed on the ward manager to take note of the nurse's views, otherwise the ward manager may become legally liable for any negligence incurred by the nurse in question.

2. The same point applies to a nurse who feels competent to be a named nurse in most situations but feels she lacks competence to plan the care of a **particular patient**. Her code of professional conduct advises her on this issue (UKCC 1992). If the ward manager, as before, fails to act on the nurse's request then the ward manager may be deemed legally liable for that nurse's potential negligence, and might also be cited as negligent by her wrongful delegation (Tingle 1993).

3. If the delegation of named nurses to patients is not correctly practised then, again, the named nurse may refuse to accept the delegation. This would occur if, for example, a nurse was allocated to a patient either in her absence, except by a mutually agreed method of allocation, or just prior to her days off or holidays. Unless there are particular circumstances, for example, in long stay units, this practice seriously inhibits the named nurse functioning satisfactorily, and she may feel the need to refuse acceptance of patients in such circumstances.

In each of the above situations **the solution is to develop an agreed system which allows named nursing to work as it is intended to work**.

Before implementing a named nurse programme on your unit, therefore, it would be advisable to receive agreement from your nurse managers on the following pattern of allocating nurses to patients.

1. Each patient is entitled to a named nurse.

2. Each registered nurse is liable to be a named nurse.

3. The nurse has the right to refuse to be the named nurse for a patient if:

- the nurse feels that she lacks the competence to provide care,

- the patient is a relative or friend,

- the nurse will be on 'days off' immediately after the current period of duty,

- the nurse will be on leave from the ward for whatever reason for the majority of the patient's projected time in that department of the hospital, and

- the nurse finds that on return to the ward from 'days off' or leave (for any reason) she has been allocated a patient who has been on the ward for more than 24 hours, except by prior agreement on allocation procedures.

On the legal risks of practising named nursing, Tingle (1993) reassures us that 'if the named nurse charter standard is introduced and operated in a reasonable manner, the risk of litigation will be much reduced'.

WHO DECIDES?

Who decides which nurse is allocated to which patient? This may depend on a number of factors.

1. There may be a wish to keep numbers balanced, with each nurse having equal numbers of patients, **or** if the emphasis is on attempting continuity of care, the decision might take workload and dependence into account.

2. The shape or design of the ward may make it very simple for the designation of patients depending on where the beds are situated.

3. The consultants attached to the ward may have a nurse or a team designated to their patients.

4. There may be a division of ward staff with teams allocated to different areas.

5. With patients in long-stay or rehabilitation units, or with repeated admission it may be appropriate for the patient to choose his named nurse.

The first question is who decides and when, and on what basis. Does the ward manager make all the decisions? This has many advantages, such as assessing each nurse's workload, and the containment of responsibility for such decisions with one person. However, the main flaw here is that the ward manager is not always available. At the other end of the spectrum, the decision could be left to the nurse who admits the patient, with the agreement that, if possible this nurse will be the named nurse for that patient. If, for any of the reasons already cited this is unacceptable then she may allocate the patient to another trained nurse. The problem here is, how does she decide which nurse to choose? She might leave the allocation to the nurses coming on at the next shift. The problem persists. Who decides and on what basis?

This programme is not designed to provide all the answers. It is designed as a deliberately simple structure so that each area can modify and elaborate on it to suit particular circumstances. On the question of allocation, the decision must rest with the ward staff, with one piece of advice. **DO NOT** make the first decision **final**. Pilot it and then discuss any problems which may have become evident, and perhaps pilot another approach and discuss it again.

Remember that poor allocation can create bad feeling and a sense of favouritism or victimisation. This will sour the ward atmosphere and have a negative effect on motivation levels and morale. It is therefore an important aspect of the programme.

THE QUESTION OF OVERALL RESPONSIBILITY

It is worth re-emphasising that named nursing is **not** primary nursing where the primary nurse necessarily carries overall responsibility for a patient's care even when she is not on duty. The named nurse is responsible for what **she does** and what **she writes**. In her absence the nurses on duty have responsibility to ensure that each patient's care and care plan is modified as necessary to meet any change of circumstances occurring during her span of duty. The named nurse, on her return, will update the care plan and sign and date it.

TO ASSOCIATE OR NOT

The associate nurse is an integral part of primary nursing. She is not, however, an essential part of the named nurse programme. The associate nurse can provide valuable support for the named nurse and the patient, but the association can only succeed on a ward where team nursing, patient allocation, or primary nursing is well established. However, if the ward management system cannot facilitate a named associate nurse on a regular basis, but rather attaches the label on a random basis, the philosophy of the associate nurse can be lost and the label becomes meaningless. This can lead to frustration and a reduced sense of job satisfaction.

TRANSFERS TO AND FROM OTHER WARDS

The simplest solution to this problem is to treat the transfer to your ward as if it were a new admission and allocate the patient to a named nurse in the usual way.

The named nurse cares for her transferred patient and plans his care from the time of transfer. She will, naturally, make close reference to the previous named nurse's care plans and records (and communicate with her if possible) and will use these as a basis of her own plans. But she builds her own plan based on her meetings with the patient and carers/relatives and all relevant information, using the named nursing programme.

Transferring the patient to another ward should be treated like a discharge with a suitable variation of the final discharge meeting to meet the individual demands of the event.

STAFF ABSENCES

In the event of staff taking unplanned absences from the ward, the patient will be notified as soon as possible. Depending on the patient's condition, his potential length of stay, and the anticipated length of absence of the named nurse, the decision will be made to re-allocate the patient into the temporary care of another staff member.

PERSONALITY PREFERENCES

This is one of the most frequently raised problems in discussions on primary nursing – what if the patient does not like the nurse, or the nurse prefers not to nurse the patient? On the latter point the question of the nurse's choice was clarified at the beginning of this chapter. The question of patient preference proves not to be a problem in the practice of primary nursing, except in very rare circumstances, for example, with ethnic differences between the patient and the nurse (Wright 1990). Any problems in patient preference is best resolved by an experienced ward manager, who will frequently find that skilled communication with the patient should resolve most problems.

PATIENT ACCESS TO NURSE DUTY ROTAS

This seems to be a popular subject in named nurse discussions. Many nurses do not agree with giving patients copies of their off-duty times because it is not necessary, and if changes occur the patient may get confused. Nurses may decide, on an individual basis, whether to tell patients their duty rota. The nurse will already have given the patient a date and time for their next meeting in writing, which obviates the need for more detailed information except in special circumstances.

It is the nurse's free choice to divulge whatever personal information she wishes on this issue.

WARD MANAGEMENT OF PATIENT QUESTIONNAIRE RESPONSES

The main fear for the named nurse, and also for the ward team about providing a patient questionnaire is the potential deluge of complaints which such an invitation may prompt. Even one complaint is an unpleasant experience, and our natural survival instincts tell us to avoid such situations.

The provision of a structure which promotes sufficient relevant communication with a patient-centred, goal-oriented approach should considerably reduce the level of patient or relative/carer dissatisfaction, and should enable **nurses to take the initiative** to respond to and resolve potential problems before they arise. The meeting structure, and the patient questionnaire, if managed correctly, should act as early warning systems for potential complaints, and should provide the opportunity for speedy resolution of them.

The Department of Health's (1994a) study of complaints found that complainants are more easily satisfied when the complaint is resolved at the first point of contact. The more people involved in the discussion, the less the complainant felt satisfied. 'It should therefore be an objective to resolve as many complaints as possible at the first point of contact. This is also cost effective for the organisation.'

But what about the nurse who is usually the first point of contact? During her discussions with her patient she will expect to hear oral complaints regularly, and is accustomed to resolving these as they arise.

However the responses in the patient questionnaire may include what seems to be a written complaint, and currently each hospital has agreed policies on dealing with these.

It is essential that the ward or unit has clear guidelines, agreed by all, as to how to handle the responses from the patient questionnaire, and, with 'more praise for good complaints handling and less blame for things going wrong' (Wilson 1994), nurses should be able to avoid:

- poor response to the complainant, leading to further dissatisfaction;

- disagreement among nurses about how to handle comments
from patients/carers;

- inappropriate or heavy handed response from hospital management.

Do **not** start the patient questionnaire aspect of the named nurse
programme without ward/hospital consensus.

MANAGING COMPLAINTS

If the response to the questionnaire implies dissatisfaction and the
nurse is unsure whether or not the patient wishes to make a
complaint, it would be advisable for her to discuss this with the
ward manager.

Fear of litigation, or of negative responses from the ward manager
may inhibit the nurse from action. However, the nurse has already
recorded notes from her meetings with the patient. These notes
should be able to identify the date and time of any expression of
satisfaction/dissatisfaction of care which the patient/carer commu-
nicates. The structured record is a safeguard.

Lloyd-Bostock *et al* have shown that, in the majority of cases,
litigation cases against hospitals do not start out as complaints
(Department of Health 1994a). Therefore, most people who make
a complaint to the hospital do not bring litigation suits as a result,
or rather, most people who bring litigation suits against a hospital,
do not initiate the procedure with a complaint. However, it must
be noted that some complainants do use the complaints procedure to gather evidence with a view to a civil claim (Department
of Health 1994a).

SUMMARY

The following points are relevant to this discussion.

1. All complainants wish to be taken seriously. Therefore a careless attitude, or a delay in response may increase the sense of dissatisfaction.

2. As many as **half** of all complaints are made by a relative, **not the patient** (Department of Health 1994a) so do include immediate relatives or carers as much as possible.

3. Lloyd-Bostock *et al* (Department of Health 1994a) have shown that hospital complaints focus on issues relating to:

   - Medical care   29%

   - Communication, behaviour and attitude   22%

   - Hotel services   22%

   - Access to treatment   19%

   - Management policy and political issues   4%

   From the above statistics it appears that the named nursing programme provides an opportunity to address a large percentage of hospital complaints.

4. It is important for the nurse to recognise the difference between a **complaint** and a **suggestion for improvement**, and to act accordingly.

5. If appropriate a simple apology may be all that is required and this can be given without personally accepting responsibility for the cause of the complaint, but rather as a representative of the unit.

6. It would be an excellent strategy to acknowledge by phone all suggestions for improvement, and even written complaints can be handled this way. 'It is an indication of tangible concern, as well as a way of exploring details of the problem and possible forms of resolution' (Department of Health 1994a).

7. It may be useful to request training on:

■ recognising the different types of complaint,

■ first line contact and handling of complaints,

■ recording of such contacts,

■ the support services available to staff who are the object of, or are involved in, a complaint, and

■ hospital policy.

4

The Structured Ward Manager's Role in the Named Nurse Programme

**Breaks with tradition – Clinical leadership – Clinical
accountability – Practice meetings – Manager's yearly plan
for practice meetings – Practice meetings as clinical audit
– Suggestions for successful change – Professional
knowledge development – Practice: the centre of
professional learning – Atmosphere as change agent –
Beware the clique – Clinical supervision – Summary of
the proposed new structure**

BREAKS WITH TRADITION

The ward manager is employed in what is increasingly becoming
a business environment, and will find few role models from her
training days who would have guided her in learning to balance
business and professional management, and still provide an
adequate degree of clinical supervision within her sphere of
authority.

Management by clinical directorates has increased the adminis-
trative role of the ward manager (Audit Commission 1991) and
reduced her opportunities to assess the quality of the work of the
staff. It requires a length of time spent working alongside them
and even then some staff have been known to be very aware of
the manager's presence and act accordingly at that time.

CLINICAL LEADERSHIP

This chapter discusses the ward manager's role in the named nurse programme. It offers the busy ward manager a means of:

- supporting her named nurses

- simple on-going clinical audit

- clinical supervision of named nurse practice

- monitoring the care on her ward

- identifying patient satisfaction of care

- keeping herself up-to-date on relevant research data

- guiding her staff towards research-based practice

- preparing for multidisciplinary care planning

- focusing on relevant staff development programmes

- targeting and resolving potential complaints.

While the supervision of nursing work and nursing staff has always been an integral part of the role of the ward manager (Luckes 1912; Prince 1984; Beardshaw and Robinson 1990), until now it has been left to the individual manager to decide whether and/or how she monitored the care on her ward on a regular basis. How many senior nurse managers could describe the methods of clinical supervision employed by the ward managers in her area?

In 1990 Beardshaw and Robinson described the very neglected subject of the management of nursing work as 'something of a "black hole" within wider health services management'.

For many years researchers have attempted to diagnose what makes a 'good' ward manager/sister (Pembery 1980; Runciman 1983) and today one can still observe a lack of structure for the ward manager's role. More often today the ward manager is away from the bedside, or even out of the ward.

The *Nursing Times* Ward Sister's Conference (Gilbert 1994) had, as its unifying theme, the 'need for ward sisters to be more assertive about their own role as managers and leaders of teams

... they should avoid becoming merely ward managers sidelined in an office. The need to show clinical leadership, to be in the vanguard in arguing the value of nursing and to make sure nurse education delivers what modern nurses need implies a substantial redefinition of the ward sister's role'.

CLINICAL ACCOUNTABILITY

The ward manager's **control** over the patients' care for which she is **accountable** is dependent among other things on her ability to coordinate and supervise the care given.

The person who monitors the named nurse's care must be eligible to judge, to educate, to advise and to monitor that care. This means that she must be competent in her speciality.

For years ward managers have recognised that the diverse nature of their role can reduce the length of time spent at the bedside and thus deplete their confidence in their clinical competence. In a study investigating the training needs of ward sisters, the sisters themselves placed clinical updating as a priority (Orme and Trickett 1983).

The Audit Commission (1992) recognises that most ward sisters/managers 'lack confidence in their own abilities to set standards or introduce methods to improve quality'.

Not only is their clinical confidence depleted but also their ability to adhere to their Code of Professional Conduct (UKCC 1992), which states that all practising nurses must 'maintain and improve your professional knowledge and competence' (Article 3), and perhaps more relevant to this chapter, 'acknowledge any limitations in your knowledge and competence and decline any duties or responsibilities unless able to perform them in a safe and skilled manner' (Article 4).

At the *Nursing Times* Ward Sister's Conference (Gilbert 1994) Betty Kershaw reminded ward sisters of the need to continue their own professional development, for continuous updating, and for adaptability.

PRACTICE MEETINGS

While the patient–nurse meeting is the core of named nursing, the monthly practice meeting provides a structured core for the ward manager to guide and supervise the named nurse programme.

James *et al* (1990) indicated that there was a 'general dissatisfaction of the nursing staff with their unit's social atmosphere. This, however, was progressively reduced amongst those staff who were given the opportunity to discuss the feedback in monthly meetings'.

Although this research looked at the social atmosphere of the working unit and the effect of meetings on staff morale, monthly meetings with an input from staff on a democratic basis can be conducive to an increase in staff satisfaction. See Figure 4.1 for an illustration of the power of practice meetings.

Practice meetings provide a bridge between the research and practice poles of nursing, which have been identified by Bendall 1975; Alexander 1983; Gott 1984; Melia 1987; Palmer *et al* 1994. This bridge is controlled by the practising nurse.

Practice meetings are held monthly and are essentially a means of providing 'professional space' (Palmer *et al* 1994) for the discussion of nursing practice. There are a variety of ways to prepare for a critical discussion of nursing practice. Some examples would be the use of articles, relevant research, text books, case studies, patient's comments, new ideas, and other ward methods, to name a few.

The following sections are sample guides for the management of practice meetings:

- 12 month planning of practice meetings (p.46),

- format of monthly practice meetings (p.47), and

- evaluation sheet for new ideas/pilot studies (p.49).

These sections may be photocopied for use in practice.

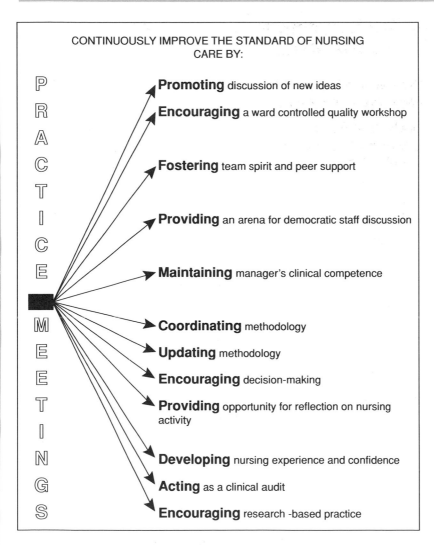

CONTINUOUSLY IMPROVE THE STANDARD OF NURSING CARE BY:

P
R
A
C
T
I
C
E

M
E
E
T
I
N
G
S

Promoting discussion of new ideas

Encouraging a ward controlled quality workshop

Fostering team spirit and peer support

Providing an arena for democratic staff discussion

Maintaining manager's clinical competence

Coordinating methodology

Updating methodology

Encouraging decision-making

Providing opportunity for reflection on nursing activity

Developing nursing experience and confidence

Acting as a clinical audit

Encouraging research -based practice

Figure 4.1 Power of practice meetings.

MANAGER'S YEARLY PLAN FOR PRACTICE MEETINGS

1. Make a list of all/most of the patients' conditions with which doctors admit patients to your area.

2. Using a physiological model, group these patients' conditions together (for example respiratory conditions), to enable staff to address the patient-centred problems associated with each group.

3. You may wish to list the groups in a sequential order to cover the 12 meetings of the year, so that the nursing care within each group, and relevant and updated research, will be reviewed at least every 12 months.

4. To promote collective ownership some units may encourage staff members to select particular areas of interest on which they would be willing to collect relevant research and pertinent data in order to prepare and present a paper for the monthly meeting. This may also encourage staff to organise and carry out pilot studies on their particular area of interest.

5. The ward manager may decide to have the sequenced list typed with date, venue, and name of presenter, and distributed to all relevant personnel.

6. A sample agenda for practice meetings is shown in Figure 4.2.

It is essential that the ward manager attends all practice meetings if she is to **maintain her monitoring competence** and her **professional knowledge**.

The time set aside for the practice meeting should be one hour. If these meetings take much longer than this, nurses and managers may become frustrated and the meeting may cease to be either productive or cost-effective.

It is the responsibility of the ward manager to promote and support practice meetings. To succeed it is essential that the atmosphere

1. Staff attendance

2. Apologies

3. Minutes of previous meeting, and any amendments

4. Report on monthly pilot studies

   • discussion
   • decision and action

5. Current topic presented

   • discussion
   • action to be taken

6. Plan for next monthly meeting

7. Date, time and venue of next monthly meeting

Figure 4.2 Sample agenda for the monthly practice meeting.

is open, non-judgemental in tone, and supportive of ideas and of a healthy questioning of the efficacy of current methods. The staff must therefore feel free to discuss what they think. No one knows everything. There is still a trend in nursing for **nurses to feel that to admit a lack of knowledge exposes them to peer ridicule** and this pressure can override their responsibility to adhere to the code of professional conduct.

PRACTICE MEETINGS AS CLINICAL AUDIT

The goal of the practice meetings is **constantly updated, research based, therapeutic nursing care**. This is a long-term and extremely challenging goal but one which can be achieved through reflective and supportive experiences promoting tolerance, and acknowledging that all knowledge is transient. Thus the maintenance of knowledge of current developments, which Vaughan and Pillmoor (1989) view as 'no longer an optional extra but an essential requirement' may be striven for, not just individually, but to meet the **collective responsibility** of each practising unit.

It is unrealistic to try to change something every month – unless the change is small. Small changes are the secret weapon in a revolution for change (Peters 1989). Do not be afraid that your pace of change is not fast enough. If, every month you succeed in making a very small adjustment in your care of patients with whatever problem is being discussed that month, by the end of 12 months, the attitude of your staff towards change will have matured, you could have developed a more cohesive, flexible, supportive team of carers who should be initiating change as a group or in sub-groups and presenting these at the practice meetings.

It will also become evident at some point as the practice meetings evolve, that the time is right to attempt greater changes. Ideally the group should be hinting at what these might be, if enough literature is available, and the group confidence has grown during the implementation of small changes. Peters (1989) says, 'Most bold change is the result of a hundred thousand tiny changes that culminate in a bold product or procedure or structure'.

At any time in the practice meeting plans, it might be useful to divide the group into sub-groups for the purpose of implementing pilots or trials of ideas. A sample form for evaluating such pilot studies is shown in Figure 4.3.

SUGGESTIONS FOR SUCCESSFUL CHANGE

Do **not** try to change care methods all at once. Successful, lasting change is best achieved when

■ Everyone knows, understands and agrees with the proposed changes;

■ The planned change can fit into the current structure;

■ The planned change will not cause uncontrolled disruption of other management/working methods;

- The change is controlled and agreed by those people who will be implementing the change;

- The surrounding services/personnel who may be affected are aware of the changes;

- The change agents work together in support of the change and communicate freely in a peer capacity about the change and its effects and any modifications required;

- The plan, its implementation, evaluation and possible revisions are all recorded – either at the time or as soon as possible after the events.

Topic:

Action taken:

Findings:

   Strengths:

   Weaknesses:

Decisions:

   Implement   _____

   Further pilot study required   _____

   Reject   _____

Comments:

Date: Signature:

Figure 4.3 Evaluation of pilot studies.

PROFESSIONAL KNOWLEDGE DEVELOPMENT

The clinical practice meeting has the potential to provide an accessible and realistic forum for solid professional knowledge development because

- It is based on current practice;

- It facilitates reflection on current practice;

- It promotes goal-oriented, knowledge-based, professional practice through an on-going learning programme;

- Each individual will bring to the meeting her own experiences of practice;

- Changes will have a practice-based platform as recommended by the Audit Commission (1991);

- Research findings can be assessed for value conflicts in the practice setting;

- Tacit knowledge in which 'we know more than we can tell' (Polanyi 1967) at long last, has a forum for visibility and clarification;

- It provides an opportunity for re-interpretation of practical experiences which, according to Mezirow (1988) is what **learning** is about;

- It provides an opportunity for on-going professional development;

- The ensuing practice will be less tradition-ridden and ritualised.

PRACTICE – THE CENTRE OF PROFESSIONAL LEARNING

Bines and Watson (1992) emphasise strongly the need for practice to be at the centre of professional learning, 'without this focus on practice it is unlikely that the skills required for competent practice will be developed. It is therefore essential that approaches which facilitate learning through practice are considered. While many courses have incorporated periods in practice in their curricula, this does not necessarily develop competence. It is not enough to be practising; being there does not equal learning. The need for a tool which practitioners can use to facilitate learning through practice is crucial'.

The successful use of practice meetings will open the door to the practitioner, rather than the researcher, to identify the need for and initiate research into particular areas, and thus the current yawning gap between nursing research and nursing practice might be reduced by the practitioners, not the theorists.

McMahon and Pearson (1991) view that 'the time when the performance of research is a fundamental component of the practitioners role' is still some time away. However those nurses who are committed to practice meetings and are confident and assertive in their practice, may yet prove that that time is not quite so far away!

ATMOSPHERE AS CHANGE AGENT

In promoting an **environment** which allows for change to occur, the right **atmosphere** is essential.

How do you produce an atmosphere? Well, how would you produce a romantic atmosphere in your home? You consider the smell, room temperature, the subdued lighting, the log fire, the music, what you wear, what you say, where you sit, and what you provide. Every reader understands how to do the above, although each will bring her own personality to bear on it. The same applies to the ward. The atmosphere or **environment** must be **worked at** so that the staff feel **safe enough** to try out new things, to break from the routine which they know so well. In order to change, **mistakes** are inevitable. **Without mistakes there can be no growth**.

A useful barometer of the success of practice meetings is the enthusiasm with which:

- The changes are implemented;

- Suggestions arise for discussion from the majority of group members;

- Healthy debate becomes a normal part of the discussion.

Be aware of the group mildly agreeing with most of the suggestions put forward – this response would suggest that the changes are merely **paper exercises**.

BEWARE THE CLIQUE

It is equally **important to recognise the 'clique' element in many nursing wards. These groups invariably retard the professional development of its members, and such group influences can be an invisible barrier to rational discussion and growth**. Their main driving force is fear of change as this will invariably reduce their control and self-protection in the ward milieu.

CLINICAL SUPERVISION

So far in the named nurse programme:

1. The named nurse has a forum for goal-directed communication with the patient/carer.

2. The named nurse plans and coordinates the patient's care.

3. The patient is involved in the planning, and in the decisions on his care.

4. The patient has an opportunity to voice his opinions on the care given.

5. The nursing care is exposed to clinical audit through the monthly practice meetings.

Named nurse's name on care plan	
Date of first meeting	
Was it within 24 hours of admission?	
Patient/nurse meeting recorded in care plan	
Achievable, realistic goals identified	
Indication of goals being met	
Patient knows his named nurse	
Patient knows the time and date of next meeting with named nurse	
Patient understands his plan of care	
I agree with plan of care	
or	
I have discussed and amended plan of care **with** named nurse	
Signature: _____	
Date: _____	

Figure 4.4 Ward manager's checklist for monitoring care plans.

This section offers the ward manager a method of clinical supervision of the nursing care on her ward without having to devote a large percentage of her time to this end.

Tingle (1993) reminds us that the ward manager 'is responsible for the named nurse and owes a legal duty of care to the patient' and Hancock (1992b) places legal responsibility for the work of the named nurse firmly with the sister/charge nurse. The named nurse programme offers the ward manager a simple monitoring routine by which she selects a small sample of care plans every week (five or six) and places her signature to signify her acceptance of the plans. Random selection might be the fairest method

Named nurse clinical supervision record sheet.			
Name of Ward:		Name of Manager:	
Patient's name	Hospital number	Nurse's name	Date

Figure 4.5 Clinical supervision record sheet.

to ensure that no one nurse is assessed more frequently than another.

This monitoring programme is designed as a cost-effective approach to supervising standards of nursing care in a busy ward environment. It also incorporates the priorities for quality improvement measures of 'patient perceptions, easily quantifiable indicators which may raise questions about quality of care, assessments of the way nursing care is delivered and of the ward environment' as indicated in the Audit Commission report (1991).

Essentially it facilitates the ward manager's need to retain overall responsibility for nursing care on a unit where individual responsibility for patients is delegated to specific nurses.

The checklist shown in Figure 4.4 may be placed in the care plan. A record of the ward manager's monitoring activity can be kept in a diary. It might be useful to use the format shown in Figure 4.5 for this purpose.

The weekly clinical supervision regime acts as

■ Support for the named nurse in her professional development;

■ A means of promoting a basic minimum standard of care;

■ A means of individual assessment of nurses;

■ A means of ensuring that practice meeting decisions are being implemented – i.e. clinical audit;

■ An opportunity for the ward manager to discuss with, and lead her staff on their development continuum in a structured way.

'The most effective supervision of nursing practice is one which shows respect for the ideas and opinions of others' (Butterworth and Faugier 1992).

SUMMARY

The proposed new structure for the ward manager in the named nurse programme should include the following features.

1. Pre-planned, pre-scheduled, routine monthly practice meetings. It is essential that these very quickly become part of the ward routine. The format should be stable, simple and easily understood with regard to not only the preparation but also the execution of its decisions. As far as possible the outcomes should be measurable.

2. The ward manager attends all of the practice meetings.

3. She monitors and countersigns at least five named nurse care plans every week, using the checklist (see Figure 4.4).

4. She records her clinical supervision (see Figure 4.5).

'It has been suggested by Platt-Koch (1986) that the goals of supervision are to expand the therapist's knowledge base; to assist in developing clinical proficiency; and to develop autonomy and self-esteem as a professional.'

In Butterworth and Faugier's (1992) discussion of the subject, clinical supervision is viewed as an 'enabling process and involves not penalties but an opportunity for personal and professional growth'. As a result, skills should be constantly re-defined and improved throughout professional life, and critical debate about practice activity is used as a means to professional development. Clinical supervision offers protection to independent and accountable practice.

5

Patients in the Named Nurse Programme

The captive audience – The new consumer – The named nurse and power transference – The power issue

THE CAPTIVE AUDIENCE

Until recently National Health care provision has been playing to a captive audience. This monopoly has encouraged the growth of a benevolent dictatorship with the main premise that providers of the service know what is best for the users of the service. The acceptance of such subservient attitudes by patients is still evident today, especially in the older generation, many of whom have been institutionalised into passive acquiescence, and are prepared to have the professionals 'do what you have to do, since you know best'! The rise of the alternative medical culture however shows the patient voting with his feet, and looking elsewhere for answers or support.

THE NEW CONSUMER

Many workers in the health service object to describing the patient as a 'customer' or a 'consumer', and I understand their views and the conflict such words provoke (Barker and Peck 1987). The reality is, however, that not only is the patient becoming a customer, but also the trend is heading toward the patient, in the future, as manager of his own personal health/financial resources, and thus may become a direct and active participant in the choice of provision, and in measuring the effectiveness of services available to him.

This concept is not peculiar to Britain. It has its recent origins in the Canadian practice of brokerage (Brandon 1989), where the patient has control of the use of services, and in the North American development of case management where a budget is allocated to a manager on behalf of a patient, for use in the provision of appropriate services to match the client's needs (Hugman 1991).

THE NAMED NURSE AND POWER TRANSFERENCE

In Britain such control of services has been based on the recommendations made initially by Griffiths (1988). The resultant potential decisions, however, which such consumers have been eligible to make to date have been greatly constrained within specific economic and social boundaries. Even the declaration that each patient is entitled to a named nurse, as a potential source of power, is frequently illusory, except where the named nurse understands the power transference which occurs once a person becomes a patient, and is mature enough to accept and allocate measures of power as a choice within the nurse–patient equation.

Nursing policy and practice will be much more rigorously assessed in the future than it has been to date. This will be stimulated by the increase of patient-led scrutiny of practice costs, litigation issues and patient-focused effective practice.

A summary of the benefits of structured named nursing are shown in Figure 5.1. The most immediate effect for the patient is that it gives him the opportunity to voice his opinions: not through advocacy, but through communication with his named nurse within a structure which provides **time** for the patient to speak.

Better communication → **More information**

→ **More control over decisions**

→ **Empowerment**

→ **Partnership in care**

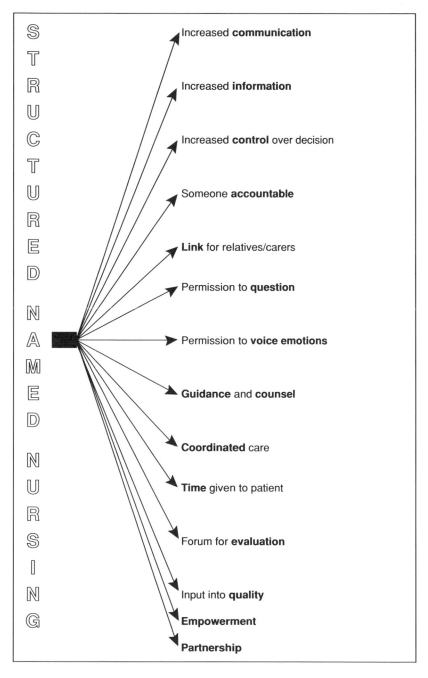

STRUCTURED NAMED NURSING

Increased **communication**

Increased **information**

Increased **control** over decision

Someone **accountable**

Link for relatives/carers

Permission to **question**

Permission to **voice emotions**

Guidance and **counsel**

Coordinated care

Time given to patient

Forum for **evaluation**

Input into **quality**

Empowerment

Partnership

Figure 5.1 Structured named nursing makes **patients** winners.

The named nurse programme also offers the patient, in the form of the patient questionnaire, a forum in writing, which is not restricted to the traditional 'Thank you for your care' or 'I wish to complain', which are usually the only two options when giving an opinion on care provision.

The patient should ensure that he receives this questionnaire and he should take the time to fill it in. It is like having the vote. Too many people do not bother to vote at elections – they decline to use the power given to them.

Perhaps the patient will return this questionnaire when he 'knows' the nurse who has asked him to do so. He might like to say what he thinks of her care, how she could improve, or what she did well.

> This questionnaire **empowers** the patient.

But, most importantly, the named nurse programme gives the patient a formal role in the planning of his care. He is no longer necessarily the passive recipient of care as the lowest in the pecking order of a dominant *vs* subservient hierarchy.

The named nurse programme, by permitting the patient to exercise 'informed consent' in his care planning, promotes the transfer of power. In today's health care environment such power can only be achieved when the nurse herself has come to recognise, understand, and begun to control the power trap which enforces itself on her working day.

THE POWER ISSUE

In order for the nurse to be in a position to give power to the patient she must first understand how she gains and retains that power.

Pearson (1992) discusses the power of the professional worker in the health care field. He points out how such theorists as Goffman (1963), Goss (1963), Field (1972) and Zola (1975) have each emphasised how professional power can be exerted to make compliance with professional values through societal pressure. He also cites Norris (1979) who provides us with one of our goals for the future of nursing, to allow our patients and their families 'to take the initiative, to take responsibility, and to function effectively in developing their own potential for health'.

The nurse exerts her control through the habits, customs and rules both formal and informal which shape the daily routine of ward life. As Hugman (1991) explains, 'Even the lack of encouragement and support may be as great a constraint for a person with a disability (whether physical or mental) as direct restraining action'.

The compliance of the patient is achieved through the knowledge that he may be totally dependent on the service for his comfort, sustenance and well-being. He is also dependent on them for recognition as an individual, for his status in the world of patients.

It is for all of these reasons that advocacy has acquired such prominence. Patient advocacy is the recognition that people may lose power when they become patients. For example, relatives and visiting times still constitute a real threat to nurses' power because they bring with them elements of life outside hospital over which the nurse has no control. Every nurse knows that she should recognise the relative or carer as a powerful force in the majority of situations on the continuum towards well-being and independence for her patient. But they threaten her control over her tightly structured environment. They have the ability to question and criticise in a way which the patient, separated from the power sources outside the hospital, would feel less inclined to voice.

The relative/carer comes between the nurse and her patient; interrupts that bond which the nurse in her systems, and with the power of control delegated to her by her institution, asserts instinctively unless she becomes aware of it through reflection on her experience and her actions.

Hugman (1991) identifies particular patient/client behaviour as resistance to the power of the nurse with its antithetical lack of personal power for the person who becomes a patient. These behaviour patterns are familiar to all nurses and are identified as uncooperative, manipulative, obstructive and ungrateful. The reader should feel free to add to this list of behaviour, descriptions which make it awkward for the nurse to exercise her institutional power and authority.

It is important for the nurse to recognise these attitudes in the context of the power struggle. This will assist her in finding the cause of the resistance and providing any clarification which may be possible.

There is a risk, with the communication promoted in this book, that the nurse will expose herself and her patient to the nurse's fallibility, even to her lack of knowledge. Why do nurses and doctors have to pretend to know all the answers? What will they lose when they admit that they do not know? This is a complex arena but the main point, for the purpose of this text, is to understand and recognise what it means to transfer such power/ authority over to the client, promoting an independence and autonomy on the patient, which, in turn, also shifts the responsibility for getting well, or for well-being, back to the patient. This, I think, is the ultimate role of the nurse. She acts to support the patient in this, if it is possible or achievable. If not, then she supports and assists the patient in retaining control over his present and future life experiences.

This power must be shifted gradually, especially when the patient expects to take on a traditional passive, non-participating role.

6

Postscript to the Unit Manager

Support or lip service? – What's in it for the unit manager? – Entrepreneurs in the workforce? – Starting with the truth – The strategy

SUPPORT OR LIP SERVICE?

In order to achieve successful implementation of a ward-based structure it is not only advantageous if ownership of the change is placed in the hands of the practitioners, but also that hospital managers understand and support the practitioners in their on-going changes to improve nursing practice and patient care. In other words bottom-up approaches to change are more successful if endorsed by top-down support with practical commitment to support the agents of change.

The main problem for the management team in supporting ward-based change is the distance created by hierarchical structures between direct patient care and the daily routine of most managers. **Commitment may be measured in relation to its clarity of vision.** One may sanction a generalised commitment to support for change. However, unless someone on the management team really understands the energy, motivation and team spirit required at the practice level, for successful implementation of a change process, and can interpret managerial commitment and support sensitively, practically, and constructively, the commitment to change may be construed at the practice level, as mere lip service, and even as hypocrisy.

WHAT'S IN IT FOR THE UNIT MANAGER?

The named nurse programme offers managers many advantages (see Figure 6.1) including a structure with a strategic direction plus feedback loops. The monthly practice meeting provides a ward-based clinical audit prompting continuous change, up-dated skills, research-oriented practice and a flexible workforce. Also included is clinical supervision of nursing care and recorded monitoring of that care. The patient/nurse meetings act as the primary building block for the named nurse, and offers a goal-orientated dialogue with the patient, as consumer. Although probably only a small percentage of patients will use the questionnaire, it is a step in the direction of patient empowerment by giving them a voice and inviting them, as important members of the multi-disciplinary care team, to comment on the quality and effectiveness of care given.

The weekly monitoring of care plans and support by management for practice meetings should not only keep standards high, but also provide a safety net for the nurse, the ward manager, and ultimately the hospital management against an increasingly litigious public. Critical assessment of practice within this ward implementation structure should develop a ward nursing team with the following characteristics.

1. They are aware of the latest research findings in their specialty.

2. They have a forum designed to maximise the implementation of relevant changes and research findings into the practice arena.

3. They permit a monitoring system which

   ■ encourages and supports implementation of new ideas,

   ■ provides a safety net against public criticism and litigation, and

   ■ promotes ongoing communication between nurse and nurse managers on nursing practice.

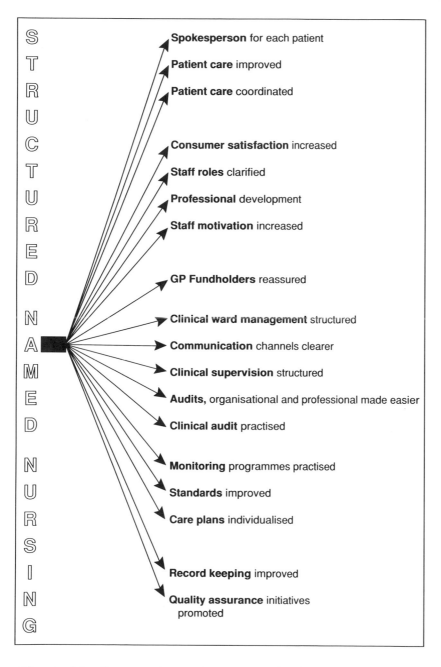

Figure 6.1   Structured named nursing makes **hospital managers** winners.

Each of the above structures which the named nurse programme addresses are intended to fit into whatever management style is operational at present. It starts with where health care is today, placing control of change in the hands of the workforce and pointing the direction of patient-focused care.

ENTREPRENEURS IN THE WORKFORCE?

The built-in record of each stage of the programme facilitates, in the long term, such organisational quality agendas as performance review measures, and fitting into an organisational audit programme. The role of unit managers is to support the named nurse programme as a bottom-up approach to change, recognising the attitudinal changes and flexibility which the manager, as role model, must not only project, but also understand, support and encourage in others. In measuring one's own attitude it may be useful to take an objective look at one's unit. *Is it a hive of innovative change agents? If not, why not*? Who are the entrepreneurs within the workforce? How often are the challenging opinions sought of dynamic nurses within the unit? Nursing is becoming a graduate profession. Is this increase in education and professional reflection evident in the activities of staff? What has been done to harness and channel the new graduate trend in nursing?

The manager should be familiar with the four structures of the named nurse programme and of the potential for a domino effect of change within units where structured named nursing is working. Although setting up the structure may only effect one change at a time, depending on what has been happening, or **not** happening in that area, a chain reaction could occur, freeing up a myriad of static possibilities.

Be alert to the possibility for growth when this is in place – and visibly encourage any progress, and tolerate mistakes as a necessary part of the change process and as an aspect of growth which has a lot to teach the group.

STARTING WITH THE TRUTH

Today's managers of health care provision are faced with a choice. It is not automatic that those who are in control today will help or be able to shape the health care environment of tomorrow. The coming scrutiny of health-care budgets will soon expose the obvious that 'when it comes to exploiting the information revolution health care is still in the Dark Ages' (Wyke 1994).

If managers choose to ignore their role as entrepreneurial interpreters of the future direction of one of the world's largest industries, the future will still happen. It cannot be stopped. It can only be ignored. However, as with all role occupants in the health care provision of tomorrow, the managers need to ask themselves whether or not they intend to **be there** in the future, and how do they plan to get there.

Those managers who do intend to hang-in and hold-on, and not just be an 'also-ran' should ensure that they have a clear picture of where health care in their unit is today not where **they would like** it to be, not where **they tell** others it is, not where **others tell** them it is, but **the truth**, unless as Jack Nicholson says in the film *A Few Good Men*, 'you can't handle the truth'.

All plans and strategies for future direction should, if they are to succeed, start from the truth of what is happening today, otherwise failure is built-in.

The overall strategic direction of the organisation relies on the quality of care provision for its long-term success. It is not enough for the managers to set a strategic direction and hope that the staff understand their part in the overall plan. The successful manager will also understand the working climate which she has created in her unit and the force fields which prompt, inhibit, prejudice or promote communication, action and initiatives from staff.

The manager may convince herself that she is open, approachable and fair and that she understands and supports her staff in realising their initiatives for change. Experience has shown that bottom-up approaches to change have a better chance for success if supported by senior management. Unfortunately the rigid bureaucracy of hospital tradition and the force fields frequently inherited by senior managers as part of the staff's interpretation of managerial decisions can present a formidable barrier to communication and mutual support. The expectations of actions by hospital managers are frequently based on force fields inherited from past managers. For staff and managers to work together towards agreed goals, it is incumbent on managers to recognise how they are perceived by their staff.

In implementing the named nurse programme, nursing staff frequently work in a stable organisation with a perception of management which controls their working lives by maintaining a system of reward and punishment where, all too frequently, praise goes to the staff member who maintains the status quo (Halek 1990). Too often systems are interpreted as being run by quick-to-blame, slow-to-praise, can't-stand-criticism guys, who only promote those who agree with them and who won't challenge them. Those for whom the light at the end of the tunnel has already been switched off! Those for whom the tunnel is the comfort zone of mediocrity and they have stopped asking 'how', and they don't know why.

THE STRATEGY

The Audit Commission (1994), addressing the NHS Trust Boards, identified three main responsibilities of these Boards as a basis for success. It emphasised the need to

- Set a strategic direction;
- Ensure . . . a system of individual accountability throughout the organisation; and
- Review the performance of the organisation as a whole.

These recommended strategies almost mirror the strategy of the named nurse programme, which sets a strategic direction, ensures a system of individual accountability, and provides a means of reviewing performance.

It also offers an answer to the 'how' question at the practice of nursing level of the organisation and as a long-term strategy it addresses the 'why'. Those who hold the purse strings are very much aware that nursing management takes a full quarter of their budget (Audit Commission 1991) and thus the financial implications of getting it wrong is a terrifying prospect. However, think of the implications of getting it right!

7

Where to Next?

Structure as springboard – Effective and economical –
Marketing confidence – Practice meetings – the multidisciplinary team – Valuing staff knowledge – From
technical competence to therapeutic expertise – Eighteen
months later! – Basic nursing techniques – Patient-centred
practice and the ward routine – Is 'routine' a naughty
word? – Time management – Communication indicators –
The development of the practice meetings – The personal
journey

STRUCTURE AS SPRINGBOARD

The purpose of adding this final chapter to the named nurse
programme is firstly to re-affirm that **this structure is designed
as a springboard from the present to the future**, it is not an
end in itself. Second, to take a glimpse of what that future might
look like for nurses, and third to suggest some small steps which
might take nursing further along the road towards the 21st century,
and what changes to this end may be identified within 18 months
of implementing the named nurse programme.

Once the named nurse programme is up and running and the staff
are taking ownership of it, the practice meetings are the main
building block for continuous change, with practitioners taking
ownership of the changes and using the other three structures
as feedback on and for change. My advice for success in the
future is to seek out the company of those who look for the right
way to do things and to avoid those who are sure they have
found it!

EFFECTIVE AND ECONOMICAL

The present shape of the National Health Service will probably alter considerably in the future. The current rigid role definitions between professional groups may be eroded and replaced with flexible multidisciplinary professionals. The nursing profession, which in many situations today, still seems to be trapped in a time warp of self-imposed bondage by rituals and routines, will face radical change towards economic, flexible, effective practice. Not only will the boundaries between professionals be blurred but also the hospital/community care structure is becoming more inter-active, less distinct.

Where is the professional role of the nurse in this? Although the future offers an opportunity to develop the scope of professional practice, it also brings with it a very real threat for the nurse as a professional hands-on care provider. Paragraph 55 of the Heathrow Debate says:

> Two other forms of substitution cannot be avoided in the scenario under discussion: replacing in a world of limited resources the expensive by an equally effective cheaper equivalent, and replacing the less effective by the more effec-tive.
>
> (Department of Health 1994b)

Is nursing today offering the cheapest method of producing the effect they achieve, and which nurses today are more effective, and which are less effective? These are deceptively simple ques-tions, and beg the following questions:

- Are you effective? What do you effect?

- How do you know whether you are effective or not?

- Is there a more economical way of producing the effect which you achieve in your work?

Perhaps it is time we all questioned our effectiveness.

The main difference between effectiveness and efficiency, with which it is often confused, can be illustrated in a discussion following a meeting: one person may say 'wasn't that an efficient meeting, so well run, so orderly and the timing was perfect'. This comment prompts another – but was it effective? What did it achieve?

MARKETING CONFIDENCE

What are we achieving as nurses? Are we effective or merely efficient? Effectiveness 'will increasingly be the key to recognition. Research-based knowledge must underpin and inform nursing practice' (Department of Health 1994b). With the increasing trend of measuring quality in relation to defined outcomes of care, the effectiveness of each person's actions will be a regular part of the measuring agenda.

The Heathrow Debate (Department of Health 1994b) identifies three main areas to which, it is felt, nurses are best suited in the future.

1. Where the nurse focuses on people, 'how they live and feel', with 'care as a process of human interaction' (para 62).

2. The role of the nurse as coordinator, key worker and case and/or care manager, including discharge planning with the elderly (para 63).

3. The role of the research-based skilled nurse practitioner (para 64).

The named nurse programme addresses each of these areas, promoting an increase in **assertiveness and expertise in what nurses do best** today, and maybe with the increase in self-confidence, take control of what we might do in the future.

Nurses are advised that in the future they will 'need to be confident in their all-round abilities and market themselves' (Department of Health 1994b). How can the named nurse programme be developed to make the journey easier?

PRACTICE MEETINGS – THE MULTIDISCIPLINARY TEAM

One step towards 2010 would be to **involve the multidisciplinary team in the practice meetings and changes**. Gradually the discussions and decisions could be made multifocal, looking at flexible, inter-professional team management of particular topics, and at the effectiveness of both the plan of care/cure and the implementation of that plan. With regard to the effectiveness of many of the present day treatments Wyke (1994) says 'the value of many other present day treatments remains obscure; indeed, in many cases, no proper study of their effects on health has ever been done'.

VALUING STAFF KNOWLEDGE

Current medical and nursing practices will be increasingly exposed to scrutiny for effectiveness and for side-effects. So also will management of nursing effectiveness such as in the questionable value for money of the huge cost of not only initial training but also ongoing training in the form of courses and study days. Frequently these study days and courses are random and there is no measure of their effect either on the nurse or of the unit's care provision. **If study days and courses were chosen in relation to decisions made at practice meetings**, with follow-up and effectiveness recorded in the minutes and change records, not only would the cost be validated but staff morale would increase as staff knowledge became valuable to the unit's effectiveness.

FROM TECHNICAL COMPETENCE TO THERAPEUTIC EXPERTISE

This emphasis on the utilisation of nursing knowledge acts as encouragement to the nurse who is struggling to **progress from technical competence to skilled expert therapeutic practitioner**, and to create a therapeutic environment which McMahon

(1991) describes as 'the interpersonal as well as the physical environment'.

As the nurse becomes comfortable with the structured named nursing format, she should reflect on her methods of communication. Communication with the patient in the structured meetings should be approached in such a way as to allow the patient to learn about himself, how he thinks about himself and his illness. This process places the nurse and patient together on a continuum towards the patient's self-assessment of his behaviour and attitudes to sickness and well-being, and is a major step in the process of therapeutic nursing (Peplau 1952; Hall 1969; Alfano 1985; McMahon 1991).

However this is not a simple procedure for the inexperienced nurse and requires skills in understanding attitude and behaviour, and in communication and empowerment.

EIGHTEEN MONTHS LATER!

This section discusses the sorts of changes or indicators of changes which should be identifiable approximately 18 months after the named nurse programme has been implemented.

These changes are not definitive or exclusive. Many wards or units may be able to identify these trends prior to implementing the named nurse programme. It may be useful for the ward manager to make a record of where she estimates her ward can be described with regard to the following pointers, before implementing the programme. An example of a measurement indication which may prove useful is the ward atmosphere scale (James *et al* 1990) which offers a baseline measure of ward social atmosphere.

BASIC NURSING TECHNIQUES

The nursing staff will have been questioning their practice at the practice meetings, using constantly updated nursing research, patient feedback, and clinical supervision. Criteria for judgement of the effect of nursing practices should be becoming a vocal and visible part of nursing discussions and decisions.

One indicator of change might be the availability of research material. Instead of being tucked away on a shelf, this material should be growing substantially in volume. It may frequently go missing as staff take it home to read. This might create the demand for a signing-out book.

PATIENT-CENTRED PRACTICE AND THE WARD ROUTINE

The goal for the future in nursing is patient-centred practice, and although primary nursing has been pointing in this direction for at least 25 years, with many countries adopting it as their aim (Hegyvary 1982), Beardshaw and Robinson (1990) still view the successful adaptation of British hospital nursing to a patient-centred practice as 'a distinctly uncertain prospect'. Thus, regardless of what the profession would like to be doing, the implementation of such a basic and obvious goal as patient-centred practice still seems to be difficult in the current hospital climate (Audit Commission 1992).

Structured named nursing gives the **patient an opportunity to begin to control the definitions of what his problems are**, rather than relying on the nurse to define what she thinks his nursing needs are according to

- Her professional competence;
- The availability of services/resources;
- The hospital policy;
- The ward routine;
- Current ward care management.

If the nurse finds that she cannot meet his needs, then, the very fact that the needs have been identified and recorded, may lead to changes in the

- Nurse's professional competence;
- Availability of services/resources;

- Hospital policy;

- Ward routine;

- Current ward care management;

based on the patient's definitions of his problems, and the nurse's understanding and recording of unmet needs.

So, while patient-centred practice is the long-term goal, perhaps the short-term goal is to make the 'routines' more patient-focused, and to provide routines which question practice and methods, and in the long term, allow the nurses in practice, to change their methods, but at their own pace, and to their particular patient/client identified requirements.

Structured named nursing is a tool which can easily fit into the routine of the present ward environment, yet it provides a stepping stone towards **breaking out** of that routine. After a year or so it should be possible to identify the patient's place in the ward as closer to the centre of the daily routine than is the current trend.

Windows of opportunity to question the ward routine for its effectiveness might be found

- In the structure/outcome of the nurse/patient meetings;

- In the patient questionnaire – the nurse's personal (and routine) evaluation questionnaire;

- In the practice meetings which will open a window to a questioning attitude;

- In the ward manager monitoring system which stimulates the professional accountability of the manager of the ward routine;

- In the clinical supervision programme.

IS 'ROUTINE' A NAUGHTY WORD

A highly routine model of nursing 'resisting patient involvement and encouraging patient conformity to the established rules' (Pearson 1992) has been identified as recently as 1992. Pearson cites McFarlane (1980) to extend the argument that 'the caring role of the nurse has been so neglected' that he says it needs 'in-depth expansion as well as the development of a nursing model of care'.

Routine is not inherently dehumanising, **we all live by routine**. How do you make a cup of tea or coffee? How do you react when someone makes it differently?

It is not the routine which is dehumanising, it is **what the routine incorporates**. Just as one routine can consistently create a fine cup of coffee, so equally another routine can consistently make a poor cup of coffee.

Another hurdle for the practising nurse is that she is trapped into relying on others to carry on her programme of care while she is not on duty. There are limits to the degree of individualisation which the plan of care can tolerate and still succeed within a hospital setting.

The more individualised the care, the more difficult it is to create continuity over a 24-hour period. Therefore, to ensure a basic standard is maintained the care requires an agreed, and easily recognised format.

TIME MANAGEMENT

From the start of discussions on implementing the structured named nurse programme, the main question might be time management. The question, 'where are we going to get the time?' may even be part of each month's discussion on changes to practice. The question might be more fruitful if asked 'how can we best manage our time? What priority indices do we use? What can be delegated or deleted? Who makes unnecessary demands on our time?'

In a busy ward environment, with traditional rigid bureaucracy, structures and habits, one indicator of change might be a more visible control over the nurse's use of her time. Breaking away from a routine based on a medically directed model of practice by recognising the influence of that routine and its power of entrapment in professional immaturity is not easy especially if the ward has a reputation for being well organised and efficient.

The relevant question is about the ward's effectiveness by its inclusion or omission of the patient's invisible needs. The very pace of the unit can be a dehumanising factor, unless the patients are involved in the pace and not approached as distractors of efficiency.

COMMUNICATION INDICATORS

These indicators might come from a variety of sources.

- *Written indicators*. After 18 months of structured patient/nurse meetings, many nurses should have developed their care plans in such a way as to reflect the patient's view and her responses, and this will be seen in more individualised care plans.

  The main problem with goal-oriented nursing care plans is in identifying what is a nursing goal. Defining nursing goals requires diagnosis, judgement and prescription.

  These activities are open to interpretation, disagreement, mistakes, confusion or inference, ridicule and risk. Such exposure can be traumatic given the frequently tightly structured nature of nursing activity. The practice meetings might, after 18 months, have reduced the trauma of peer ridicule in making these decisions.

- *Peer suppport and development*. Another indicator of change might be recognised in nurses' communication among themselves. Of all the professions, nursing is perhaps the one most practised in a mutually supportive capacity. We need each other! As a ward group we are only as good as our weakest peer. Even though one nurse can provide an excellent supportive environment with high levels of hidden agenda nursing, the nurse following her to that patient, either on the same shift, or the next one, can very easily demolish all the invisible empowerment structures so carefully placed by her predecessor.

Once the ward recognises its developmental level with regard to therapeutic nursing care, then the starting point for progression is clarified, and the ward can begin to develop as a group.

■ *Nursing demand for skills training*. Implementing the patient/ nurse meeting structure should slowly begin to identify individual and collective requirements for training on a variety of communication skills including informative counselling skills, bereavement counselling skills, and complaints handling skills, to name but a few. If by the end of 18 months of practising the named nurse programme, such demands are not being made, one might question the nurses' commitment to the programme.

■ *A nursing voice*. Ward agreement on patient care based on relevant research, successfully implemented in practice, should produce a body of opinion which is clearly identifiable and coherent. The nursing staff who practise in this way should begin to find increased recognition of nursing opinion in the multidisciplinary setting, and should be able to recognise the effect of knowledge-based power within the multidisciplinary groups.

■ *Patient satisfaction*. Patients and carers should be making more comments on their care. Although not all comments will be positive, the increased communication between patient and nurse should heighten the overall sense of satisfaction with care given.

THE DEVELOPMENT OF THE PRACTICE MEETINGS

In the first year or so the practice meetings will probably be involved in the technical competence and scientific knowledge aspects of practice because these are

- Highly visible;

- Easily discussed;

- Easily measured; and

- Competence is achievable even for the inexperienced nurse.

Technical competence can be described as being skilled at the ward routine, fast and efficient, displaying competence in all technical nursing tasks, and being a good medical assistant.

As the practice meetings become second nature, and the staff have progressed as a group, then gradually the group should be progressing to the more therapeutic aspects of nursing practice. A good start on this road would be to attempt to define, as a group, the main differences between technical competence and therapeutic practice.

There is an old saying that 'You cannot see until you see'.

Colliere (1986) explains that the reason why the care component, which is the baseline of holistic practice, remains an invisible aspect of nursing work, is that 'those who occupy themselves with it within the workforce are socially unconsidered, powerless and marginalised in terms of their perceived usefulness'.

Meerabeau (1992) leaves us with the reassuring thought that the expert practitioner not only utilises research-based knowledge but 'creates new knowledge' and that 'practitioners' knowledge is a largely untapped resource'.

Therefore, another fund of knowledge for the practice meeting agenda is already sitting around the table. The art is to learn to express this tacit knowledge, and learn to learn from each other.

Tick ONE box in each section	Never heard of it	Heard of it but don't understand it	Understand it but don't know how to do it	Know how it should work but awkward in practice	Can practise it sometimes	Natural part of my daily patient care routine	Promotes the practice with the team
Score	0	1	2	3	4	5	6
Provides an aura of healing							
Promotes patient empowerment							
Self-awareness through reflective practice							
Empathy and respect for each individual							
Fully sensitive to unvoiced needs/ fears/ wants							
Skilled listener							
Skilled communicator/ counsellor							
Promotes open relationships							
Able to cope with patient involvement within defined limits							
Alert to dehumanising effects of ward routine							
TOTAL							

Figure 7.1 Therapeutic practice self-assessment scale (continued on p83).

What does your score mean?

SCORE

60	What can I say?
50–60	Excellent!
40–50	Where most experienced nurses should find themselves
30–40	Keep up the good work – going in the right direction
20–30	Find a good role model
10–20	Find a seat in the library – keep reading
0–10	Don't believe you!

Figure 7.1 (continued)   Therapeutic practice self-assessment scale.

Why does one nurse have a different approach to her patients than another even with a strict routine? Why does a nurse work more easily with nurse X than nurse Y? The reason is that each nurse has her own personal model of nursing in her head (Reilly 1975; Wright 1990). This is an instinctive model, and few nurses could either recognise or describe their personal model, yet it dictates how they approach and care for their patients. It also indicates where each nurse may be on a technical competence–therapeutic nursing continuum and may explain why some nurses seem to 'fit-in' to the team easier than others.

One way to measure your success on the journey to professional, competent, therapeutic practice might be to use the self-assessment scale shown in Figure 7.1.

The difference between therapeutic and holistic nursing has been described by Hockey (1991): 'Therapeutic nursing can now be explained as the practice of those nursing activities which have a healing effect or those which result in a movement towards health or wellness. It is important to emphasise that both 'healing' and 'health' must be regarded as multidimensional, and should include physical, emotional, spiritual, mental and environmental

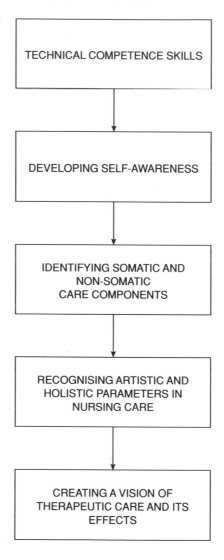

Figure 7.2 A guide for professional development.

considerations. Such a wide interpretation allows therapeutic nursing to be offered as part of terminal care. . . .holistic nursing, the care of the 'whole person', is a necessary but not a sufficient condition of therapeutic nursing'.

In exploring the nurse's and the unit's attitude to the care component of nursing work, a plan of professional development may be useful, using the headings in Figure 7.2 as a guide.

References

Alexander MF (1983) *Learning to Nurse. Integrating Theory and Practice.* Edinburgh: Churchill Livingstone.

Alfano GJ (1971) Healing or caretaking – which will it be? *Nursing Clinics of North America*, 6:273.

Alfano GJ (1985) Whom do you care for? *Nursing Practice*, 1(1):28-31.

Astley J (1992) Knowledge and Practice. In: Binnes H and Watson D (eds) *Developing Professional Education.* Buckingham: The Society for Research into Higher Education and Open University Press.

Audit Commission (1991) *The Virtue of Patients: Making Best Use of Ward Nursing Resources.* London: HMSO.

Audit Commission (1992) *Making Time for Patients: A Handbook for Ward Sisters.* London: HMSO.

Audit Commission (1994) *'Trusting in the Future' – Towards an Audit Agenda for NHS Providers.* London: HMSO.

Bailey JT and Claus KE (1975) *Decision Making in Nursing: Tools for Change.* St Louis: CV Mosby.

Barker I and Peck E (1987) 'Thinking it Through'. In: Barker I and Peck E (eds) *Power in Strange Places*. London: Good Practices in Mental Health.

Beardshaw V and Robinson R (1990) *New for Old? Prospects for Nursing in the 1990s.* London: King's Fund Institute.

Bendall E (1975) *So you Passed, Nurse.* London: Royal College of Nursing. Quoted in Palmer A *et al* (1994).

Bines H and Watson D (1992) *Developing Professional Education.* Buckingham: Society for Research into Higher and Open University Press. Quoted in Palmer A *et al* (1994).

Bradley J and Edinberg M (1990) *Communication in the Nursing Context.* Norwalk, USA: Appleton and Lange.

Brady E (1992) Where is the named nurse for all? *Nursing Times*, 88(24):14.

Brandon D (1989) The courage to look at the moon. *Social Work Today*, **20**(50):16–17, 139.

Burnard P (1989) *Counselling Skills for Health Professionals.* London: Chapman and Hall.

Butterworth T and Faugier J (eds) (1992) *Clinical Supervision and Mentorship in Nursing.* London: Chapman and Hall.

Castledine G (1993) New BJN initiative to close the theory/ practice gap. *British Journal of Nursing*, **2**(9).

Cole A (1993) Name check. *Nursing Times*, **89**(14):30.

Colliere MF (1986) Invisible care and invisible women as health care providers. *International Journal of Nursing Studies*, **23**(2):95–112.

Davies B (1985) The clinical effect of interpersonal skills: the implementation of pre-operative information giving. In: Kagan CM (ed) *Interpersonal Skills in Nursing.* London: Croom Helm.

Department of Health (1991) *The Patient's Charter.* London: HMSO.

Department of Health (1994a) *Being Heard.* The Report of a Review Committee on NHS Complaints Procedures, Wilson A (Chair). Camberley: Department of Health.

Department of Health (1994b) *The Challenges for Nursing and Midwifery in the 21st Century. The Heathrow Debate.* London: Department of Health.

Druker PF (1967) *The Effective Executive.* London: Heinemann.

Field D (1972) Disability as a Social Disease. In : Friedson E and Corber J (eds) *Medical Men and their Work.* New York: Aldine Atherton.

Gilbert J (1994) For all they are worth. *Nursing Times* Ward Sisters Conference. *Nursing Times*, **90**(17):18.

Goffman E (1963) *STIGMA.* Harmondsworth: Penguin Books.

Goss MEW (1963) Patterns of Bureaucracy among Hospital Staff Physicians. In: Friedson E (ed) *The Hospital in Modern Society.* Toronto: The Free Press.

Gott (1984) *Learning Nursing.* London: Royal College of Nursing.

Griffiths R (1988) *Community Care: An Agenda for Action.* London: HMSO.

Halek C (1990) Myth or reality. *Nursing Standard*, **4**(37):47.

Hall LE (1969) The LOEB centre for nursing and rehabilitation. *International Journal of Nursing Studies*, **6**:82–83.

Hancock C (1992a) The named nurse concept. *Nursing Standard*, **6**(17):16–18.

Hancock C (1992b) The named nurse in perspective. *Nursing Standard*, **7**(1):39–42.

Hayward J (1975) *Information – A Prescription against Pain.* London: Royal College of Nursing.

Hegyvary S (1982) *The Change to Primary Nursing.* St Louis: CV Mosby.

Hockey L (1991) Forward. In: McMahon R and Pearson A (eds) *Nursing as Therapy.* London: Chapman and Hall.

Hugman R (1991) *Power in Caring Professions.* London: Macmillan Education.

James I, Milne DL and Firth H (1990) A systematic comparison of feedback and staff discussion in changing the ward atmosphere. *Journal of Advanced Nursing*, **15**:329–336.

Kramer M (1974) *Reality Shock.* St Louis: CV Mosby.

Lawler J (1991) *Behind the Screens. Nursing, Somology and the Problem of the Body.* Melbourne: Churchill Livingstone.

Lewis FM and Batey MV (1982) Clarifying autonomy and account-ability in nursing services, part 2. *Journal of Nursing Administration*, **12**(10):10–15. (From a study of hospital complaints (clinical and non-clinical), by Lloyd-Bostock and Mulcahy *Report to ESRC – Citizen Grievance Initiative – Complaints about Hospitals* (unpublished), cited in Department of Health (1994a).)

Luckes EC (1912) *Hospital Sisters and their Duties.* 4th Edition. London: Scientific Press Ltd.

Luin K (1947) Group decision and social change. In Newcomb TM and Hartley EL (eds) *Readings in Social Psychology.* New York: Holt, Reinhart and Winston.

Manthey M (1980) *The Practice of Primary Nursing.* London: Blackwell Scientific Publications (Reprinted (1992) London: King's Fund Centre).

Meerabeau L (1992) Tacit nursing knowledge: an untapped resource or a methodological headache? *Journal of Advanced Nursing*, **17**:108–112.

Melia K (1987) *Learning and Working – The Occupational Social-isation of Nurses.* London: Tavistock.

Mezirow J (1988) *Transformation Theory.* Adult Education Conference Paper, South East (cited in Ersser, 1991).

McFarlane J (1980) *The Multi-disciplinary Team*. London: King's Fund.

McMahon R (1991) Therapeutic Nursing: Theory, Issues and Practice. In: McMahon R and Pearson A (eds) *Nursing as Therapy*. London: Chapman and Hall.

Naylor MD (1990) Comprehensive discharge planning for hospitalised elderly. A pilot study. *Nursing Research*, **39**(3):156–161.

Naylor MD and Shaid EC (1991) Content analysis of pre- and post-discharge topics taught to hospitalised elderly by gerontological clinical nurse specialists. *Clinical Nurse Specialist*, **5**(2):111–116.

Nightingale F (1859) (republished 1980) *Notes on Nursing*. Edinburgh: Churchill Livingstone.

Norris CM (1979) Self care. *American Journal of Nursing*, **79**(3):486–489.

Orme L and Trickett M (1983) Identification of the training needs of sisters and charge nurses. *Nursing Times*, **79**(24):29–32.

Ottoway RM (1976) A change strategy to implement new norms, new style and new environment in the work organisation. *Personnel Review*, 5(1):13–18.

Palmer A, Burns S and Bulman C (eds) (1994) *Reflective Practice in Nursing. The Growth of the Professional Practitioner*. Oxford: Blackwell Scientific Publications.

Pearson A (1985) *The effects of introducing new norms in a nursing unit: An analysis of the process of change*. Unpublished PhD Thesis. Goldsmith College, University of London.

Pearson A (ed) (1988) *Primary Nursing*. London: Chapman and Hall.

Pearson A (1992) *Nursing at Burford. A Story of Change*. London: Scutari Press.

Pearson A and Vaughan B (1986) *Nursing Models for Practice*. London: Heinemann.

Pembury SE (1980) *The Ward Sister – Key to Nursing*. London: Royal College of Nursing.

Peplau HE (1952) *Interpersonal Relations in Nursing*. New York: GP Putman and Sons.

Peters T (1989) *Thriving on Chaos. Handbook for a Management Revolution*. London: Pan Books Ltd.

Platt-Koch LM (1986) Clinical supervision for psychiatric nurses. *Journal of Psychological Nursing*, **26**(1):7–15.

Polanyi M (1967) *The Tacit Dimension.* London: Routledge & Kegan Paul.

Prince J (1984) *Miss Nightingale's Version of a Nursing Profession.* Interim Report. London: Royal College of Nursing.

Reilly D (1975) Why a conceptual framework? *Nursing Outlook,* 23(9):12–20.

Royal College of Nursing (1993) *Refusal to Nurse, Guidance for Nurses.* London: Royal College of Nursing.

Runciman L (1983) *Ward Sisters at Work.* Edinburgh: Churchill Livingstone.

Salvage J (1988) *Facilitating Model-based Nursing.* Unpublished paper. Gateshead: Nursing Models Conference.

Salvage J (1990) Promoting good practice. *Nursing Standard,* 4(41):52–53.

Thompson DR (1989) A randomised control trial of in-hospital nursing support for first-time myocardial infarction patients and their partners – Effects on anxiety and depression. *Journal of Advanced Nursing,* 14(4):291–297.

Tingle J (1993) Legal and professional implications of the named nurse concept. *British Journal of Nursing,* 2(9):480–482.

Turrell EA (1986) *Change and Innovation. A Challenge for the NHS.* London: Institute of Health Services Management.

UKCC (1992) *Code of Professional Conduct for the Nurse, Midwife and Health Visitor.* London: UKCC.

Vaughan B and Pillmoor M (eds) (1989) *Managing Nursing Work.* London: Scutari Press.

Wilson A (1994) In *Being Heard.* London: Department of Health.

Wilson-Barnett J (1978) Patient's emotional response to barium x-rays. *Journal of Advanced Nursing,* 13(2):215–222.

Wilson-Barnett J (1988) Patient teaching or patient counselling? *Journal of Advanced Nursing,* 13:215–222.

Wright S (1986) *Building and Using a Model of Nursing.* London: Edward Arnold.

Wright S (1989) *Changing Nursing Practice.* London: Edward Arnold.

Wright S (1990) *My Patient my Nurse. The Practice of Primary Nursing.* London: Scutari Press.

Wright S (1991) Facilitating Therapeutic Nursing and Independent Practice. In: Pearson A and McMahon R (eds) *Nursing as Therapy.* London: Chapman and Hall.

Wright S (1992) Should nurses wear name badges? *Nursing Standard*, **7**(3):28–30.

Wright S (ed) (1993) *The Named Nurse, Midwife and Health Visitor*. London: Department of Health.

Wyke A (1994) The future of medicine. *The Economist*, **19 March**:3–18.

Zola IR (1975) Medicine as an institution of social control. In: Cox C and Mead A (eds) *A Sociology of Medical Practice*. London: Collier-Macmillan.

Appendix

The Named Nurse:
Implications for Practice

This appendix is an extract from *The Named Nurse: Implications for Practice*, Issues in Nursing and Health No. 14, published by the Royal College of Nursing, the world's largest professional union of nurses, 20 Cavendish Square, London W1M 0AB. Telephone 0171 872 0740.

TO ACT AS A NAMED NURSE YOU NEED TO HAVE:

■ the freedom to exercise accountability and autonomy in your practice, within the boundaries of your professional knowledge (UKCC, 1984);

■ complete managerial and educational support so that you are empowered to practise in this way;

■ the confidence and interpersonal skills to form the necessary relationships with your patients, their carers and the multi-disciplinary team;

■ support in monitoring, maintaining and developing your standards of practice;

■ a working environment with the agreed proportions of qualified and support staff to deliver this approach, (RCN, 1992a);

■ opportunities for continued professional development and support;

- a manageable caseload of patients determined by:

  your own abilities and experience;

  the needs of the patients;

  your approach to nursing care;

  the geography/locality of the working environment;

- the opportunity to give enough direct patient care to enable you to form a therapeutic relationship with the patient, and to enable you to manage, coordinate and delegate care;

- the ability to help other nurses to develop their named nurse approach;

- the ability to work in partnership with other nurses, acting on their behalf when necessary. Never fall into the trap 'You are not my patient I cannot help you';

- awarenesses of different ways of organising nursing care. These have been summarised by the Royal College of Nursing (RCN, 1992b)

REFERENCES

RCN (1992a) *Skill Mix and Reprofiling: A Guide for RCN Members*. RCN: London.
RCN (1992b) *Approaches to Nursing Care*, Issues in Nursing and Health No. 13. RCN: London.
UKCC (1984) *Code of Professional Conduct*. UKCC: London.

First published in 1992 and reprinted with minor amendments in January 1996 (ref NPC/6/94).

Index